ROBERT SCHLEIP

With Johanna Bayer

FASCIAL FITNESS

How to be resilient, elegant and dynamic in everyday life and sport

lotus
publishing

First published by Riva Verlag, rivaverlag,de. All rights reserved. This English language edition published in 2017 by Lotus Publishing, Apple Tree Cottage, Inlands Road, Nutbourne, Chichester, PO18 8RJ

Important Note
This book is intended for learning purposes only. It is not a substitute for individual health counselling or medical advice. If you wish to seek medical advice, please consult a qualified physician. The publisher and the authors cannot be held liable for any adverse effects which are directly or indirectly related to the information contained in this book.

Editing: Caroline Kazianka
Cover design: Maria Wittek with Mary-Anne Trant
Cover pictures: Vukašin Latinovi
Models: Daniela Meinl, Markus Rossmann
Layout and setting: Meike Herzog with Mary-Anne Trant

Printed and bound in India by Replika Press

British Library Cataloguing-in-Publication Data
A CIP record for this book is available from the British Library
ISBN 978 1 905367 71 9

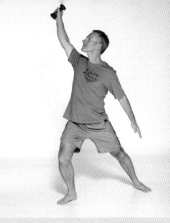

CONTENTS

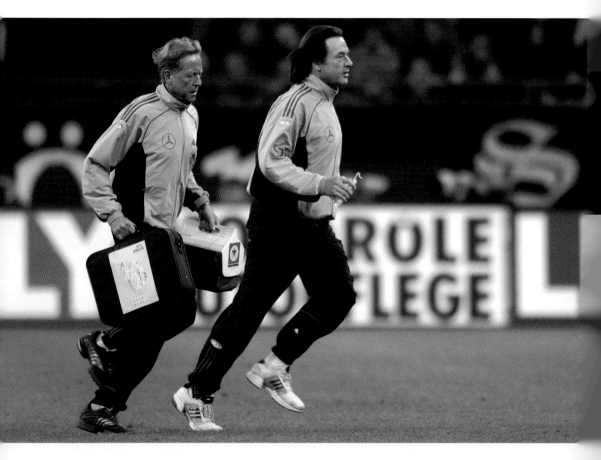

Klaus Eder (left) preparing for immediate action.

FOREWORD

by Klaus Eder

The invitation to write a foreword to a book about my favorite subject, fascia, is simply too tempting to pass up. I couldn't resist the opportunity to support a book written by my colleague and close friend Dr. Robert Schleip, whose work I admire and very much appreciate, and who shares my fascination with fascia.

The results of his research work, accompanied by his involvement in physiotherapy, have enabled him to make fascia an important part of science, as well as for sport physiotherapists, and in manual therapy techniques. I can't tell you how excited I am that he now brings this knowledge to a wide range of readers in this easy-to-understand book.

My life as a physiotherapist working with athletes spans several decades. Since 1988 I have been working with the German national football team, and in this role I have been able to treat the players during seven world championships. From 1990 until 2012 I was also in the fortunate position of working with the German Davis Cup tennis team as their physiotherapist.

The way I diagnose and treat athletes is accomplished using just my bare hands, and I get to know the consistency of most of the athletes' muscles and fascia intimately. Similarly, I know only too well about the dramatic personal challenges players face when they have to retire temporarily or permanently as a result of injury or overused muscles. I am certain that fascial tissue is always affected. In most cases, I am able to reduce the severity of the pain and reduce the time that the athletes are absent from their chosen sports.

What helps me the most under these circumstances is my knowledge of fascial anatomy and the experience as a physiotherapist that I have been able to gain over many years. However, the way I and other therapists practiced in this field was for a long time based more on intuition and experience than on sound knowledge.

The fundamental change came as a result of the work of Dr. Robert Schleip. With their experiments, he and his colleagues at the University of Ulm have added a whole new basis to the understanding of fascia. They showed that fascia can harden the muscles independently and that this can also happen in connection with stress.

As a manual therapist I can locate such hardening with my hands and fingers when examining athletes and patients; however, I often had to hold back with explanations, as I did not have any—I only had my senses. When talking to orthopedic surgeons and medical authorities, I quickly realized that they had very definite opinions about the origin of these lumps, and these opinions did not fit in with my intuition as a practitioner. Those discussions proved to be far from easy.

I am therefore very pleased that Robert Schleip received the prestigious Vladimir Janda Award for Musculoskeletal Medicine in 2006 for his experimental work, especially since I completed an apprenticeship with Janda himself. Prof. Vladimir Janda, the renowned scientist and neurophysiologist from Prague, was one of the first who pointed out to me, and to other pioneers in the field of today's sports physiotherapy, how important the fascia is for healthy body movement and how well it responds to treatment. This fact stands out and can be observed not only with my top athletes but also with those at amateur level who we have examined and treated for many years at our Eden Reha treatment center in Donaustauf in Southern Germany.

I especially welcome that with this book a fascia oriented training becomes accessible to anyone, whether professional or amateur athletes, and that the function of the fascia in the body is explained in an understandable way. This specific fascial fitness training, which Robert Schleip and his colleagues have developed in recent years, has a very high potential in my view.

It would make me very happy if this book could help more people have fun and success when exercising, without getting hurt or having to rely on therapeutic help from me and other knowledgeable fascia colleagues. Better still, this doesn't mean that we as sports physiotherapists will be made redundant, but thanks to the work of researchers like Robert Schleip our work will become easier in the future.

Klaus Eder
Donaustauf, August 2014

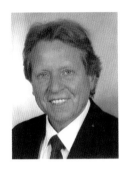

▥ Klaus Eder

is a physiotherapist and has worked for many years with top athletes and Olympians who practice many different kinds of sport, such as the German national football team and the German Davis Cup tennis team. He runs a practice in Donaustauf/Germany for physiotherapy and remedial gymnastics, along with an affiliated rehabilitation clinic called Eden Reha for sports and accident injuries. Eden Reha also offers ongoing training for physicians, health professionals, and physical education teachers, covering topics such as sports physiotherapy and fascia therapy.

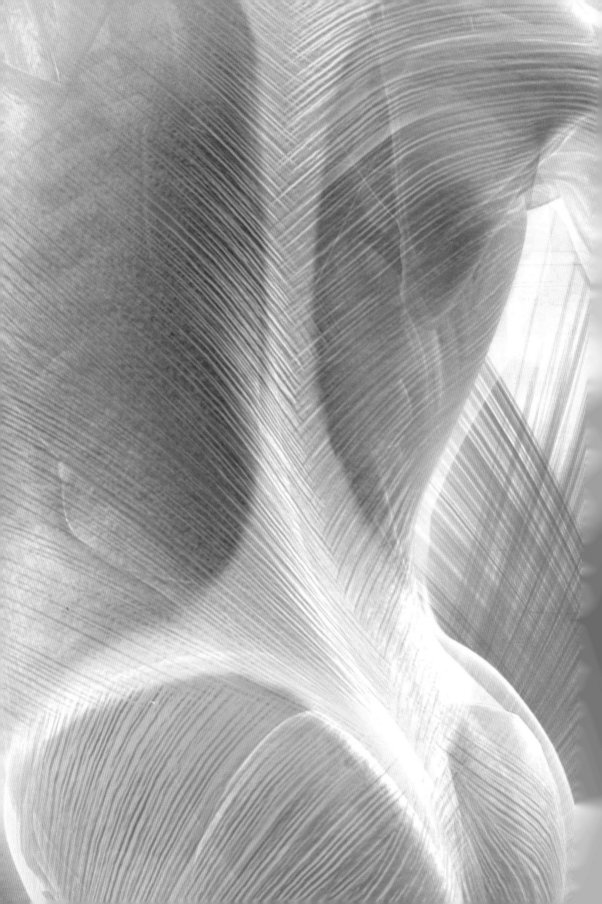

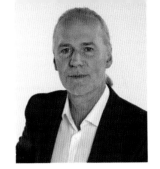

Why You Need to Exercise Your Fascia

I am fascinated by fascia (pronounced: fashia). Fascia is more commonly known as the soft tissue component of the connective tissues that run through the entire body as a covering and connecting network. It gives form and structure to our bodies. This material and its characteristics are so interesting that I changed my field of business from that of a therapist to that of a scientist. I wanted to understand the role that fascia plays when we move our body and what its real impact on our body and psyche is. Meanwhile, it became obvious to me that the importance of the fascia cannot be overstated and that we would all benefit from becoming more conscious of the influence that the fascia has on everyday life, and on sport especially.

The full meaning and complexity of this is what I would like to explain in this book. Even though the fascia has been on the sidelines for such a long time, the medical profession, coaches, and physiotherapists probably knew about its existence and function.

Historically, chronic back pain has been treated with common medications and operations. When sportsmen stagnated after long training, physiotherapists tried to alleviate pain and tension by focusing on muscles, nerves, bones, coordination, and strength; the fascia was not seen as an independent contributor. Research has significantly changed this way of thinking during the last few years: fascia has now been acknowledged and understood to be an important factor in musculoskeletal dynamics, rather than being an inert packing organ as previously thought.

Much of the existing knowledge about fascia had to be reviewed, and this even created a paradigm shift. For example, the delayed onset muscle soreness observed after heavy exercise originates less from the muscle tissue itself but comes mainly from the fascial envelope which surrounds the muscle; back pain often does not result from vertebral or intervertebral disc degeneration but from the fascia. Sports injuries are not necessarily muscle injuries but are more likely to be injuries of the fascial components. Nowadays, the fascia is considered to be one of our most important sensory organs. The connective tissue even sends signals to the brain—the heart of our consciousness. All body movements are codetermined by sensors in the fascia; if these fail, the human body loses its ability to control its movements. The list of these new realizations is enormous and is updated almost daily with information from all around the world.

Sports injuries are most common in ligaments, joint capsules, and tendons, and also fascia connective tissues. See how Holger Badstuber, number 28 from Bayern Munich, tears his ligament in the right knee.

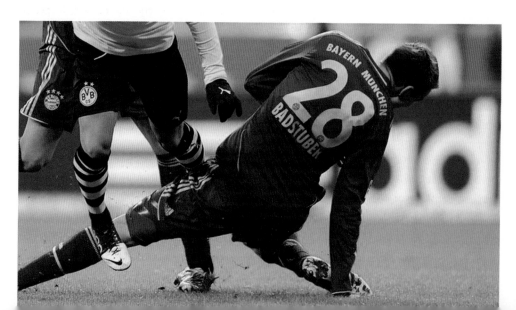

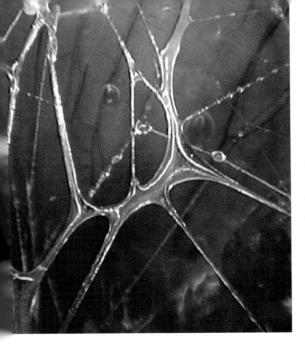

The concealed network: fascia. This unique microscopic image was taken by French surgeon J.C. Guimberteau.

New information emerges from medical or biological research, physiotherapists, and other practitioners. I worked as a body and movement therapist before I entered this field of science, so it is very important for me to connect theory and practice.

In 2009 the Fascial Fitness Association had already begun to adapt the many discoveries relating to the fascia into a training program with the goal of purposefully strengthening, stimulating, and maintaining the fascia. Today the network of fascia researchers, sport scientists, and movement therapists, who use and develop this specific fascia training, stretches around the entire globe.

There are already hundreds of books and training programs available, all making more or less the same promises: increased energy, improved body strength, greater endurance, a more beautiful body, and better mobility, health, and well-being. If someone says: "We already do everything possible," I would understand that very well; and if someone says: "Why should I change my method of training? I am happy with the way I exercise," I would understand that too, as the key thing that athletes above all know is that what counts ultimately is to exercise in the most effective way.

In the case of fascia, a component unknown until now comes into play. Purposeful fascia training can optimize the potential of training achievements and promote an increase in newly gained efficiency. It also encourages pain-free everyday life, provides relief from stiffness, and most of all is easy to incorporate into a training program. This means that fascia training does not have to replace any of your current training programs, but instead should supplement them. It enriches them with a certain element that has been missing up until now. For many decades the emphasis in sport science and training teachings has been on strength, endurance, and coordination: the focus has been mainly on muscles, cardiovascular function, and neuronal control, with very little consideration of the fascia.

Many training programs stress that they *do* train fascia, but this is only partly true—frequently the programs are not efficient, as fascia needs its own impulses and specific movements. In common, fixed, and stereotypical programs, these particular impulses are usually absent, or arise only coincidentally and without coordinated dosage. In comparison, athletes who train for a marathon of course also train the muscles; however, their capacity for weight lifting will not be improved as much as in a specialized muscle training. Thus specific training is the key to achieving total optimization. Nowadays, we know about the enormous importance of the fascia for the functioning of our muscles and their optimal coordination—but also that the fascia needs a special kind of stimulation. This knowledge affects the training concepts that have undergone several modifications over the years.

After having previously trained individual muscles, we are apparently now paying more attention to muscle groups and functional movements—and today something new is emerging: training should cover the entire fascial network and its long chains in the body. The condition of the fascia influences healing of injuries as well as recovery after training and competition. It also determines much more—and this is what you will discover in this book.

The addition of fascia training can put a finishing touch to your personal exercise program, which means that you do not need to do additional exercise programs or change your training program at all. The proposed exercises can be easily integrated and will seamlessly provide care and maintenance of the fascia network in your body.

The exercises should stimulate the connective tissue, regenerate it, and keep it vitalized and supple; thus you can train your muscles even more effectively, your movements will be more fluid and elegant, and your stamina will also increase. As fascia training increases the capacity of tendons and ligaments, it: (a) avoids painful friction in hip joints and spinal discs; (b) protects the muscles from injury; and (c) keeps the body in shape, because it produces a more youthful and taut stature. These aspects are particularly important in everyday life, and also with increasing age. Fascia training is surprisingly uncomplicated: 10 minutes twice a week is sufficient, special clothing or equipment is not required, and the entire program is simple and suitable for daily use and for all ages and levels of training.

The advantages of fascia training for sport and in everyday life are quite simply:

- Your muscles work more efficiently.

- It shortens the recovery time after heavy exercise, and so you will be ready for the next exercise much faster.

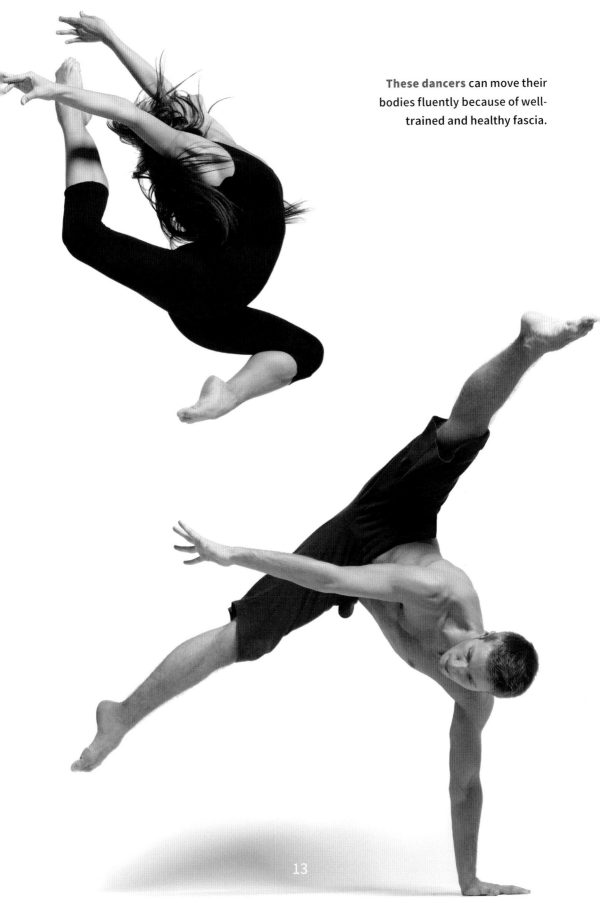

These dancers can move their bodies fluently because of well-trained and healthy fascia.

- Your athletic performance increases.

- Your movement and coordination improves.

- Your movements appear more elegant and less stiff.

- Your posture and body shape are resilient and more youthful.

The exercises I have designed for fascia training are adjustable for various connective tissue types and as we age, which is common to us all, regular fascia training should be an important part of our daily routine. Fit fascia keeps you in shape, and with the right training you can stay youthful and taut for a lifetime. So, to keep fit and feel in good shape, you should exercise your fascia regularly. In everyday life there are also other effects that concern the fascia. Many people are familiar with common ailments such as back pain, shoulder and elbow problems, neck tension, headaches and foot problems. The medical profession is increasingly recognizing that the condition of connective tissue plays an important role in all these syndromes, and that disturbances in the connective tissue can even be the cause. Problems such as shoulder stiffness (frozen shoulder), and lower back pain can often be reduced or completely eliminated with fascia-related treatments and training programs.

A JOURNEY TO THE UNKNOWN WORLD OF FASCIA

With my experience as a body therapist, researcher, human biologist and teacher, I see the fascia and its significance in many different perspectives. I use it in my scientific work in the training and further education of physicians, physiotherapists, surgeons and osteopaths. I also understand what fit fascia means to me and my body personally. When I get up in the morning, or when I'm relaxed or stretching. Sometimes, after a strenuous day, I walk around the corner to the climbing frame in the park and stretch my joints to the maximum – to the delight of the children and neighbors – who see a 60-year-old man working out on a playground. In the morning I'll walk barefoot to feel my body and adjust my senses for the day, and while working, when I have to sit for long periods, I will interrupt the rigid posture with small exercises. In my busy life as researcher, teacher and author, it would be impossible for me to maintain an efficient lifestyle without caring for my body and using fascia training.

I hope you – through this book – will experience and feel the same benefits in your body that I do. So I invite you to accompany me on a journey to the hidden structures that we can all benefit from.

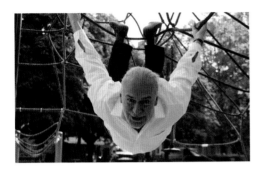

After a long working day, there is hardly anything more refreshing than swinging and tumbling around like a monkey in a playground near my apartment in Munich.

I am convinced that the function of the fascia is not only of interest to athletes, trainers and instructors, but also for readers who simply want to achieve a satisfying, fit feeling in the body and movements. This program and knowledge is especially relevant to people with pain, or older people who are looking for a meaningful, easy training regime and information to guide them. Practical tips are available in the section on diet and healthy lifestyle.

Initially, there are some chapters explaining the fundamentals together with anatomical and physiological details. However, these are simply to help with understanding the principles of fascia training that go beyond normal muscle and strength development, and have a lot to do with the properties of the tissue.

On our journey into the new world of the fascia you will learn a lot of which you are at present unfamiliar. So first, I'll help you get an overview of the properties and functions of the fascia before starting the exercises. You will benefit so much from the training and gain some new knowledge for your everyday life.

Above all, fascia training should be fun, as sensory pleasure is for many reasons, essential in our exercises. It is now time to launch our expedition with the prospect of harmony in our own body and movement.

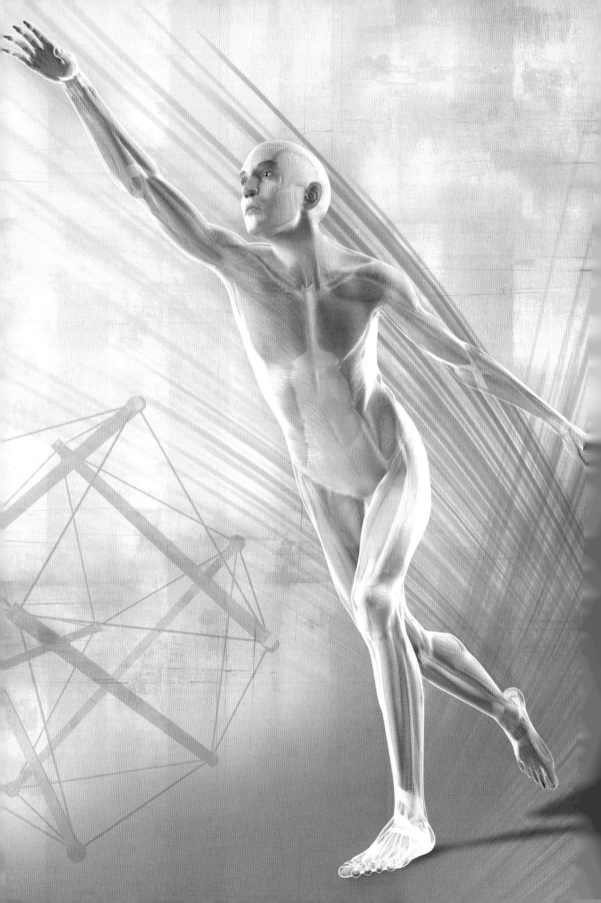

CHAPTER 1

Fascia and Connective Tissue —What Are They?

Before you exercise, you should learn more about fascia and the importance of the connective tissue in your body. The connective tissue is amazingly diverse and has features that affect the entire body. In this chapter I will give you an overview of the different types of fascia and their characteristics; you will see that the basic functionality of the connective tissue is the same for almost all of these types. In addition, the connective tissue runs throughout our whole body and is linked with various organs.

All this has implications for the type of training that my colleagues and I have developed: these exercises will be introduced in Chapter 3. The attributes or features of connective tissue are even more important when one considers that they are related to pain, as well as to certain diseases or functional limitations that vary when we age and can even affect our mental health. For this purpose the science of fascia will also be investigated.

If you would like to gain maximum benefit from your workout, the following paragraphs are therefore important. Those of you who are in a great hurry may wish to skip this chapter and scroll to the exercises in Chapter 3. In a quiet moment, however, you should come back and read this information, as you will benefit even more when doing the exercises and perhaps gain some insights into ways of adapting your daily routine.

FRESH FASCIA

At some time or another, most people will probably have had a piece of fascia tissue in their hand, usually in the kitchen while cutting meat. Since we like to eat the muscle meat of animals, we often get to see the associated fascia, which traverses the meat as fine marbling and is visible as a white layer. In general, the butcher or chef will cut away the tendons and the white layers; however, depending on the type of meat and the dish being prepared, they are sometimes left in, as they release flavor and fat. If, for example, you like to have a nice, crispy crust on your roast pork, then you leave a thick piece of abdominal fascia, including fat, on the roast. In typical roast beef that is cut from the loin you can see a part of the great back fascia of the animal, as shown in the picture—it is carved ready for frying. The fascia that you see here is muscle fascia, but there are also other types of fascial tissue.

PRIMARY SUBSTANCE WITH MANY FEATURES

Fascia essentially consists of the primary substances of life: protein and water. The texture of the tissue depends on the function it serves and on its location in our body. The types of fascia and its many functions are so varied that this can prove confusing to non-professionals. Until recently, even experts were not united in their point of view on fascia. However, doctors, physiologists, and anatomists have been aware that broad fascia sheets, tendons, and ligaments, the fascial envelopes encasing our organs (such as the kidneys or heart), the ultra-thin layers around the muscle bundles and our joint capsules are all made of the same material. They are also in agreement that all the subcutaneous fat, the loose, reticulate abdominal tissue, and even the cartilage and adipose tissue have essential construction and operating principles in common.

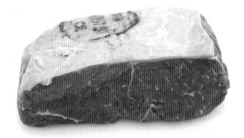

Actual fascia: typical roast beef, inside finely marbled with fat and connective tissue. The white layer is on top of a piece of large back fascia.

THE COMPONENTS OF FASCIA

Actually, all the connective tissue can be seen as a universal building material in our body, in other words fibers in a network which is sometimes fixed, sometimes loosely knotted, and also filled with some amount of liquid. This network can be both extensible and tight, tensile and tear resistant, and soft and loose; however, it always consists of the same components in different proportions—collagen, elastin, and an aqueous or gel-like ground substance.

At the first Fascia Research World Congress in 2007, the founders (of whom I am one) decided to build upon the established term "connective tissue": the connective tissue of the musculoskeletal system as well as the fibrous tissue around the inner organs we designated henceforth as fascia. We also wanted to keep all of the connective tissue features in mind. Our team thus attempted to combine the knowledge of doctors, physiologists, biologists, orthopedists, anatomists, along with that of physiotherapists, manual therapists and naturopaths.

Nowadays, fascia researchers around the entire world regard connective tissue as a specialized organ—a system that permeates the whole body and has both general and some very specific tasks.

They use the terms fascia and connective tissue largely synonymously, and the same reasoning will be adopted in this book. However, not all anatomists and physicians see it that way.

By the expression "connective tissue" an academic anatomist or a physician usually include bone and cartilage, and they therefore consider the terms connective tissue and fascia as not identical. However, this book adheres to the modern notion that "fascia" is synonymous with what is meant in ordinary language by "connective tissue".

Collagens, as part of the fascia, play an important role—they consist of fairly densely packed fibers that literally give the human body and all vertebrates their shape. They are therefore referred to as *scaffold proteins or structural proteins*.

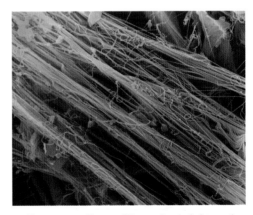

Collagens: collagen fibers viewed through a scanning electron microscope.

Collagens are the most common body proteins, with a share of 30%. They truly are a primary substance—even our bones originally developed from collagen fibers. In the womb, the embryo initially produces collagen; minerals, such as calcium, are then incorporated between the collagen layers. This is how hard bones develop from soft fibers.

There are 28 different types of collagen, four of which are very common. They have interesting mechanical characteristics: they are easily extensible, yet very tear resistant—their tensile strength can be greater than that of steel!

Elastin is the second-commonest structural protein found in fascial tissue. Its name actually suggests its most important feature: elasticity. It can stretch more than collagen and still return to its original shape. Under tension it may expand to more than 150% of its original length before, when overloaded, it finally tears.

The extensibility property is important for organs that are mechanically stressed or have to change their shape: for example, the bladder alternately filling and emptying. Thanks to the high proportion of elastin, these organs can extend and contract again like a rubber ball. Our skin, which stretches naturally when we move, contains elastin.

CONNECTIVE TISSUE CELLS

Both of the fibrous proteins collagen and elastin are produced by cells in the fascia, the actual connective tissue. These fibroblasts, sitting in the network of the fascia, actually produce the fibers of connective tissue in the amounts needed in the corresponding organ.

Fibroblasts also respond to external stresses—when you train a lot and develop strength, fibroblasts produce more fibers that help the growing muscle. The connective tissue cells regularly replace the fabric, albeit rather slowly: within a year, about half of the fascial tissue in the body will be replaced. As well as being necessary structural proteins, the connective tissue cells produce enzymes and messenger substances that fibroblasts interact with; using these mediators, they also influence the immune system. This liquid substance including its lymphocytes, immune cells,

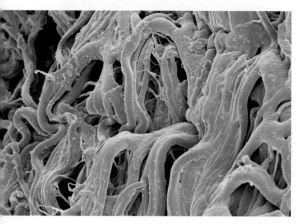

Elastin fibers of the aorta.

and various other substances is collectively called *ground substance* by experts in this field.

The connective tissue cells and fibers are surrounded by liquid in which other substances float—this mixture of fibers and ground substance is called the matrix.

The liquid portion of the ground substance consists of water and sugar molecules that bind various materials and cells together. The matrix plays a crucial role in the nutrient supply of connective tissue and the organ to which the tissue belongs. Later this subject will be revisited, when the

deeper secrets of the fascial physiology will be discussed from a scientific perspective.

It is important to note that the matrix in these different connective tissue types hosts large quantities of immune cells, lymphocytes or fat cells, nerve endings, and blood vessels, and that the water content of the matrix varies.

Water is crucial as a medium for cellular metabolism. As a consequence, various techniques used to treat fascia focus on the water content and on the exchange of fluid, and we will come to that later. Jointly responsible for the water content is

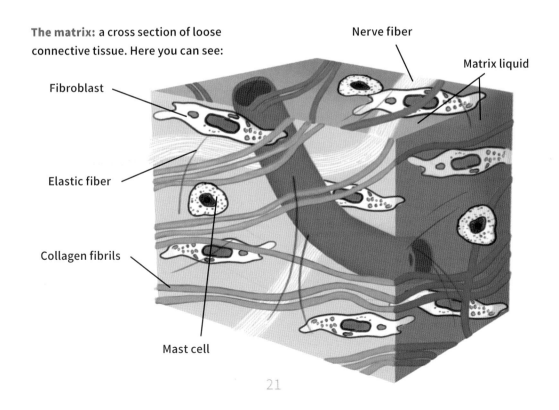

The matrix: a cross section of loose connective tissue. Here you can see:

Fibroblast

Elastic fiber

Collagen fibrils

Mast cell

Nerve fiber

Matrix liquid

a very important component of the matrix: hyaluronic acid, which chemically speaking is a polymer of sugar molecules. Hyaluronic acid is produced by the connective tissue cells; it is viscous, despite good flow properties, and forms the synovial fluid in the knee, shoulder, and hip. As hyaluronic acid is an excellent carrier of water, it plays an important role in the liquid content of the loose types of connective tissue; much of this material can also be found in the intervertebral discs. Hyaluronic acid accumulates plenty of water between the collagen and elastin fibers in the skin, and creates a plump, wrinkle-free complexion around the face. This substance is therefore very popular with the cosmetics industry: hyaluronic acid is processed into creams and preparations, and cosmetic surgeons inject it to enhance the lips.

TYPES AND FEATURES OF CONNECTIVE TISSUE

The astonishing ubiquity of fascia in the body corresponds to its different types and tasks; the following tissue types can be roughly distinguished.

● Loose, Fibrous Connective Tissue

Fibrous connective tissue contains quite a lot of ground substance, specifically liquid, but also connective tissue and

collagen and elastin fibers. It is arranged in the form of a soft, coarse mesh.

Gaps in the abdomen around the organs are filled with loose connective tissue which protects, stabilizes, and cushions the organs. The connective tissue also has very important functions for the metabolism and provisioning of the internal organs.

Loose connective tissue plumps our skin in the lower layers and includes hair follicles, sweat glands, blood vessels, and many nerve endings, as sensors receptive to pressure, touch, movement, or temperature. Typical of loose connective tissue is its wealth of immune and lymphoid cells and the fact that within it, as well as in the skin, many nerve endings, motion sensors, glands, or other cells can be found. This type of tissue forms the highest proportion of connective tissue in the body.

● Elastic Connective Tissue

There is a higher proportion of elastin in elastic connective tissue. This type of tissue can be found in organs that are often stretched: around the bladder, the gall bladder, the aorta and the pulmonary system.

Parallel, Dense, Fibrous Connective Tissue

Parallel connective tissue, with its very high proportion of collagen, forms the tendons, the ligaments, the solid capsules around the organs (such as the kidneys) or the pericardium, and all the thin layers surrounding the muscles. The fibers are aligned parallel to each other, pointing in the direction in which stress takes place, for anatomical or physiological reasons. Their parallel arrangement enables them to resist very strong tensile forces.

Irregular, Dense, Connective Tissue

In contrast, there is less ground substance and very little elastin in *irregular connective tissue*, but you will find many fibers, especially thick collagen bundles. This kind of tissue forms the linings of the brain and the lower skin (dermis); it is able to withstand high stretching forces and stresses in multiple directions.

Fibers are arranged in the direction of the different tension forces to which they are exposed. It is possible for several directions of tension to exist, which is why irregular connective tissue is referred to as multidirectional. The connective tissue cells are sandwiched between the characteristic fibers, and the liquid content is lower than in other fascial tissues.

The Grapefruit Principle: Fascia Keeps Everything In Shape

Virtually all organs are surrounded by connective tissue; the whole body is permeated by it, in various surface layers as well as in the deeper layers. To illustrate how fascia keeps the whole body in shape, my colleague Thomas Myers uses a vivid picture of a grapefruit.

The pulp of a grapefruit is enclosed in small detachments of white skin, and on the outside it is again surrounded by a solid white skin that fits snugly to the peel. If one were to remove all the pulp and leave only the white skin, one could reconstruct the entire fruit and its form, on the basis of this structure alone.

Similarly, this applies to the fascia and the human body: it is possible to see how the person looks, on the basis of just the connective tissue, without the meat and the bones. The same does not apply, however, to the skeleton.

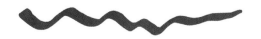

● **Reticular Connective Tissue**

Reticular connective tissue consists of a type of collagen that can form very thin fibers. It is typical of the connective tissue of the spleen, lymph nodes, and thymus, and is commonly found on freshly healing scars.

● **Special Connective Tissue**

Adipose tissue, cartilage, and the gelatinous substance of the umbilical cord are also a kind of connective tissue, referred to as *special connective tissue*. However, adipose tissue contains less ground substance and less collagen. Its specialized cells, the adipocytes, store not only fat but also water; these fat cells are surrounded by elastin. Fat has a surprising number of functions in the body: it stores energy, insulates against cold, secretes hormones and neurotransmitters, is very metabolically active, cushions organs (e.g. kidneys) and joints (e.g. knees and heels), and forms typical parts of the body, such as the thighs, buttocks, or female breasts.

During the process of aging, the proportion of water in the connective tissue decreases and the collagen fibers become increasingly matted.

Connective Tissue: Numbers and Facts

● Each person carries between 18 and 23 kg of connective tissue.

● It stores a quarter of the total amount of water in the body.

● It provides cells and organs with food.

● It responds to stress and strain, and adapts accordingly.

● It slowly renews itself constantly: after one year, about half of the collagen fibers will have been replaced.

THE NEW VISION OF OUR BODY

At present, anatomists from around the world specializing in fascia research, including Carla Stecco of the University of Padua, are operating on the basis of new representations of the body. These representations show the fascia and its body-wide network; for example, the subcutaneous fascia layer is shown tightly surrounding our body like a diver's wetsuit.

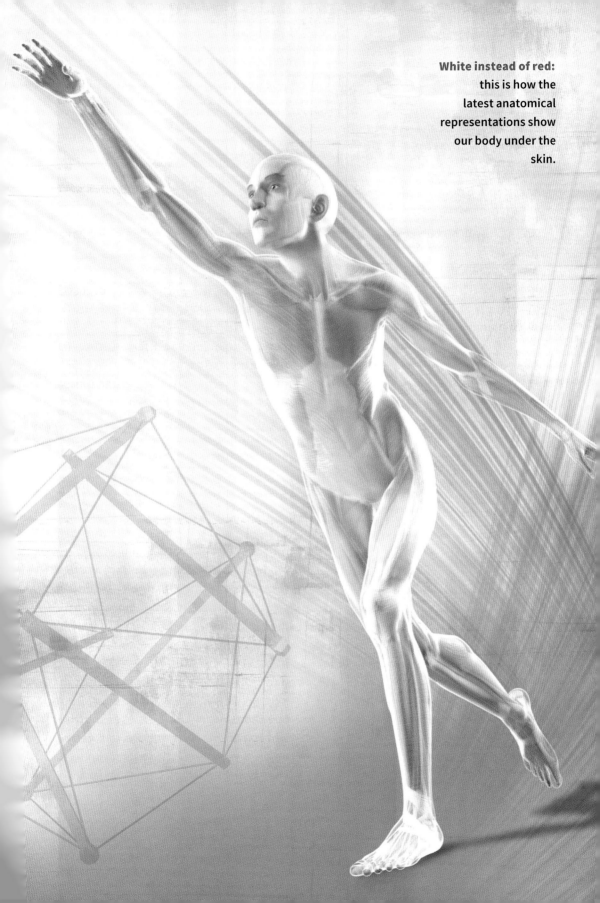

White instead of red: this is how the latest anatomical representations show our body under the skin.

THE FOUR BASIC FUNCTIONS OF THE FASCIA

The list of different connective tissue types might appear confusing at first glance, but four basic functions can be recognized (see image):

- **Shaping:** wrap, cushion, protect, support, give structure.

- **Movement:** transfer and store power, maintain tension, stretch.

- **Communication:** receive and forward stimuli and information.

- **Supply:** metabolize, transport fluid, carry food.

Since the various functions almost always occur together, complement each other, and are mutually dependent, they are seen as a kind of continuum. That is why they are represented by a circle—you will encounter this icon often in this book.

The four basic functions are therefore associated with each type of fascia or connective tissue, no matter which body part or organ it serves. Only the proportions and priorities shift: some parts of the muscle fibers contain more water and serve as suppliers, while others have less water. The tendons, for example, have virtually no functionality as suppliers. All fascial tissue, however, sends signals (it contains receptors and sensors), and also supports body movement.

Shaping and movement work purely on the mechanical attributes of the material. Fascia has mechanical and static responsibilities in the body: it provides structure for body shape, for tension in the muscles, and for movement of the limbs and their support, protection, wrapping, or padding. These tasks were recognized by anatomists in the Middle Ages, but for a long time they assigned the responsibility of actions mainly to the muscles, bones, and other organs, whereas connective tissue was basically associated with more inert material, such as the hair and nails.

A Continuum with Four Dimensions:
As discussed above, there are four
basic functions of the fascia, which are
provided by the fascia to the whole
organism.

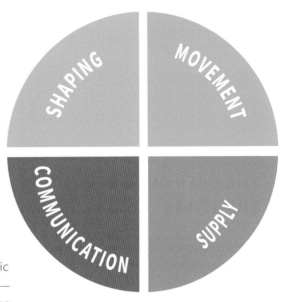

We now know that this is not always the case, because the other two basic functions—supply and communication—almost always operate at the same time. These functions are physiological benefits of living tissue; moreover, through the omnipresence of connective tissue surrounding each organ, they are indispensable for the whole process of cell metabolism in the body, for the inner perception of movement and body activity, and for the transmission of many signals throughout our body.

Incidentally, the earliest recognition of the physiological functions of connective tissue can be traced back to the late 19th century. However, it has only been in recent years, since around the 1960s, that these functions have been systematically explored. The knowledge about connective tissue has now changed dramatically from its initially being considered as a rather inert packing material, to its recognition as a supporting tissue for suitable organs, and even as an indispensable sensory organ.

Of particular importance are the physiological benefits of the connective tissue around the organs and under the skin. This tissue allows the metabolism of cells and organs, and is a medium through which lymph, blood vessels, and nerves can run; water and nutrient exchange takes place here, and there are many immune cells present as well.

Physiologists nowadays consider the general metabolic function of the connective tissue as one of its central tasks. Since the loose connective tissue runs like a network under our skin throughout our body, researchers see it as a communication phenomenon: if the supply network is disturbed or damaged at some point, there will be body-wide responses, as well as stress responses in the connective tissue.

A later section about the science of the fascia will delve deeper into this fascinating topic. You will also read more about the four basic functions in the discussion of the four dimensions of fascia training in Chapter 2.

THE DEEP CUTS OF SURGEONS

Professor Werner Klingler, with whom I work in fascia research at the University of Ulm, is a senior physician in anesthesiology. He is in the operating room almost every day, which resembles a high-tech workshop, with advanced endoscopes and many monitors on which doctors can observe processes inside the body during operations. From older surgeons he knows that previously doctors acted quite courageously and freely when operating inside our bodies. When they operated in the abdomen, gall bladder,

or cecum regions, they made long and deep cuts to reach the organs, and the fibrous pad was moved aside, severed, or cut away.

This was done out of necessity—surgeons simply wanted to get to the area of interest in order to work there in the best way possible. The inconspicuous filling tissue played only a subordinate role. The organs were exposed and operated on; the surgeon then sewed up the abdominal wall, and often took pride in the beautiful outer seam. The surgeon recognized that they had thereby destroyed sensitive tissue inside and caused scars and adhesions, which permanently affected the operated organ and its supply—but there was no other solution.

Visible scars on the abdomen are something to be avoided nowadays. Only gradually, thanks to the advances of technology, has it been discovered that smaller scars and the least possible injury to the internal abdominal cavity (even if "only" the fill tissue was affected) were significantly better for patients: they had less pain, the wounds healed faster, and there was less damage and reduced after-effects'. This was so self-evident that a set of special procedures was developed, which is now known as *keyhole surgery*—operations using small cameras, optical instruments, and microsurgical devices, which allow smaller openings of the skin and the body. Surgeons refer to these procedures as *minimally invasive*.

Visible scars on the abdomen are something to be avoided nowadays.

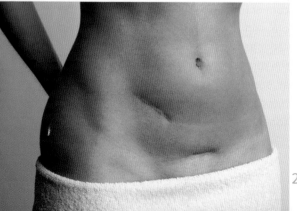

Keyhole surgery leaves only very small incisions and interventions, particularly in the inner tissue. Many studies have confirmed that when there are fewer cuts in the connective tissue and less scarring, then the wound healing process is better, the patient's experience less pain, and the recovery period is shorter. However, surgeons are not quite there yet. On the one hand, it has been found that minimally invasive procedures leave smaller scars to the skin and interfere cosmetically less, which is attractive to the patient (does anyone want a long scar on their stomach?). On the other hand, it also means that surgeons have to try to find more and more inconspicuous entry points which are far away from the original site of surgery. Depending on how the target organ is reached, the surgeon still has to cut through fascial tissue—sometimes even to a greater extent than in the past when the cut section lay directly above the organ. In an effort to penetrate at the most unobtrusive locations, the cut the surgeon has to make with his instrument may even be bigger than before.

As a result, whole layers of fascia now become more separated from each other: cuts and injuries pass horizontally through the connective tissue, whereas in the past the operational procedure used to be a vertical cut. It seems the new approach is not without its problems. It has become even clearer that surgery has to be executed as gently as possible because of the connective tissue, but there is still no universal method indicating how best to achieve this.

HIGH PERFORMANCE: FASCIA AND THE MOVEMENT OF OUR BODY

The connective tissues in the musculo-skeletal system enable our body to perform, both mechanically and physiologically, at a top level. The fact that we can move at all is unequivocally due to the fascia. Each muscle, each fiber bundle, and even each individual fiber is covered in thin fascial layers. These wrappings transfer the force of the muscle fibers, move the bundles of these fibers, and actually allow the muscle to work smoothly.

Tendons—tight fascial tissue—ensure the transfer of power to the bone. Tendons and tendon sheaths therefore also belong to the fascial structure of the muscle. Most muscles are connected by tendons to bone attachment points. In addition, long interconnections of fascial muscle units link up several body parts to each other. This occurs over long distances in our body, from the feet over the back to the head, or along the sides of our body.

A Work Unit: Muscle and Fascia

Muscles are composed of hundreds of fibers packed into tight bundles. Each bundle is wrapped in a thin fascial layer. This whole structure is again enclosed in an outer muscle fascia, which ensures that the muscle retains its shape. Beneath the smooth surface of the outer muscle fascia is a pad of softer tissue; this loosely embeds the muscle fibers.

Muscles: muscles consist of thousands of fibrous structures.

Epimysium: the outermost fascial sheath of muscle maintains the muscle shape.

Fibre bundles: thousands of fibers form dense bundles.

Perimysium: the fiber bundles are each wrapped in connective tissue.

Endomysium: thin connective tissue layer around individual muscle fibers.

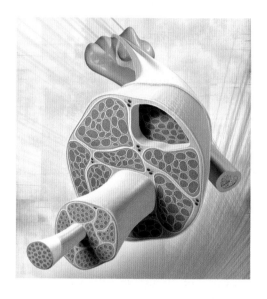

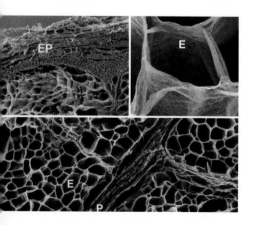

Connective tissue sheaths in a piece of lean meat seen under the microscope. Japanese researchers have dissolved red muscle tissue in caustic soda, so that just the honeycomb cases remain: top left is the epimysium; top right is the endomysium, which wraps a single muscle fiber. The lower image shows a cross section through the inside of a muscle. In addition to the abundance of endomysium (E), you can see the perimysium (P), which wraps the different muscle fiber bundles and also separates these bundles from each other.

▨ Dissected and Ignored

The muscle fascia suffered the same fate as the inconspicuous supporting tissue in the abdominal cavity: for decades only little attention was paid to the thin covering layers of connective tissue. Instead, the focus of anatomists was diverted to the eye-catching red lean meat and its visible function under the skin. On their dissecting tables they neatly peeled away everything that was white on the skin and muscles (the connective tissue), and pulled the red meat free and described its form and function. Of course, they knew and saw that all the muscles were completely wrapped in and permeated by connective tissue. At best, however, the professionals paid attention to the thick tendons, ligaments, and flat fascia which visibly connect the muscles to the bone. The consequences of this neglect have now become obvious.

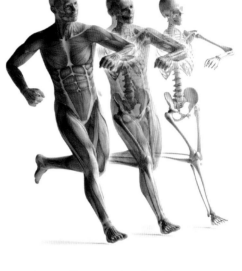

Muscles and bones – but hardly any associated connective tissue: a typical study on the anatomy of human movement, around the connective tissue.

Even today anatomical illustrations and studies of musculoskeletal systems essentially show the skeleton and muscles; anatomy atlases are therefore full of parcels of red muscle—but the associated connective tissue is hardly shown. Only a few major fascia leaves are visible, which are regarded as distribution centers, such as the large back fascia. Even the excellent standard works of anatomy devote only a few pages or foot notes to connective tissue. Incidentally, a crucial element is situated right next to the bone: a fibrous tissue layer, or what doctors refer to as the *periosteum*. The bones, like all organs of the body, are wrapped in a fascial envelope. Think of the image of the grapefruit: everything is encased. Tendons are often not attached to the hard bone, but to its outer skin, or periosteum.

THE INFORMATION CENTER: FASCIA AS A SENSORY ORGAN

Within the fine, thin, and thicker layers of fascia in and around the muscles run all the necessary nerves and blood vessels that supply the muscle. An abundance of receptors send and receive information to and from the muscle and forward this information to the brain. These receptors are nerve endings of various types; they transmit their information into the central nervous system and communicate details about stretching, movement, the position of the muscle in question, the organ, and the body part. Specifically, these nerve endings are:

● Pacinian corpuscles

● Ruffini corpuscles

● Golgi receptors

● Interstitial receptors

Medically all four types belong to the category of mechanoreceptors—these are sensors that register motion, changes in position, pressure, shear motion, or stretching. They specialize in different qualities of stimulus and intensity.

Pacinian corpuscles are programed to react to rapid pressure changes, to vibration, or to sudden impulses. These particles need dynamic alternations in motion or force. They will cease to respond if there is no change in stimulation for several seconds or longer.

Ruffini corpuscles specialize in long, alternating, and sustained pressure, and in rather quieter, steady stimuli, such as a massage or slow stretching.

Golgi receptors are unresponsive to passive movement stimulation; they only react when the stretched muscle fibers are active at the same time. They are situated in or near the tendons and are able to reduce muscle tension when the tendons are under high strain. In this way they protect the tendons and the joints from being overloaded.

Interstitial receptors are connected to the autonomic nervous system, which controls unconscious processes and movements, such as digestion. In addition to pressure and shear motion, they can signal pain and temperature; they are also the most common type of receptor.

All four types of receptor contribute to the so-called ability of *proprioception*, the self-perception of position and movement in space. It was already previously known that such proprioceptive sensors exist, especially in the deeper layers of connective tissue of the skin and also in the joints. This seemed logical, as the skin is an organ of touch and is subject to various forces, and because the joints are often exercised. Physiologists and neurologists were not surprised by the existence of stimulus detectors.

What is new is that these sensors also are present in all fascial tissues and constantly send signals about their condition to the central nervous system. Amazingly, they are far more numerous than the nerve fibers that cause muscle movement, namely motor neurons: nerves such as the sciatic nerve consist of almost three times as many sensory neurons as *motor neurons*. Therefore, human movements seem to depend mainly on the sense of movement initiated through the nervous system, instead of by triggered muscle actions.

Furthermore, as physiologists found out only recently, the number of different sensors and nerve endings in the fascial components of a muscle exceeds by far the number of sensory neurons of the muscle itself. This is especially true for those who report pain—pain arises primarily in the fascia and not in the muscle fibers. We will return to this important information later. Several years ago, the discovery that our lumbar fascia is covered with pain sensors shed new light on the chronic, unexplained back pain that many people suffer from.

▦ The Wiring of the Nervous System

The new discoveries in physiology have completely changed the image of connective tissue: specifically, the fascia of the musculoskeletal system is now considered in its own right a sensory organ and body-wide information system. Because our brain seems to rely on these continuous stimuli, it constantly anticipates and builds upon the wealth of information that it constantly receives from the fascia.

The self-perception of the body is of fundamental importance, even for seemingly simple activities such as standing upright. The sense of movement is even called the "sixth sense," but is more technically known as *proprioception, sense of movement*, or *motion perception*.

This inner perception is mainly supplied by the fascia and connective tissue around the organs, because they contain nerve endings, receptors, and sensors; these furnish information about the position and location of the organs in the area, and about their activity and their movements, through pressure and touch. Information about strain and stress is also provided through joint actions. The fascia is therefore an extended part of the brain and the nervous system, which controls movement.

Ian Waterman—
The Man Without Any Body Feeling

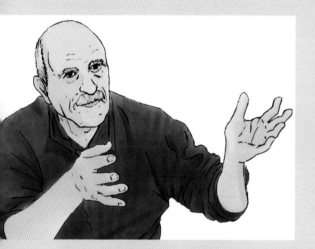

There are certain rare nervous diseases where specifically proprioception is lost. Such patients (of whom there are very few in the world) are not paralyzed, but yet are unable to move normally because they have lost their "sixth sense," namely the sense of movement.

The cause of this loss of motion perception is usually a viral infection, which leads to false reactions of the immune system. The immune system then destroys the precise nerve pathways that inform the brain about what the muscles, tendons, ligaments, and joints do. The consequence is a total lack of sense of movement within the body, something that is normally automatically and continuously processed by our brain. The sensations of pain, heat, and cold will remain intact, and motor neurons are not affected, so that movement is possible— the muscles can be activated, although more in a clumsy manner. Patients can, for example, sit in a wheelchair and tense their muscles, but they are not able to get up on their own or walk. It is a loss of the sensation of motion, which is communicated by the nerve endings in the fascia. With this disease as a starting point, neurologists have been able to measure the real importance of this "sixth sense" for the sensory control of movement. The Briton Ian

But the connection of fascia sensors for the autonomic nervous system is interesting. It explains, for example, why the treatment of fascia through massage or manual therapy has effects which can only be accounted for by focusing on the autonomic nervous system: the subjective feeling of heaviness or lightness in a body part, warmth, a feeling of relaxation in the muscle, lower blood pressure, increased heart rate, a slowed pulse, or bowel movements. Because these activities are regulated by the autonomic nervous system, it seems that manual treatment, such as in massage, reaches the sensory motion sensors in the fascia, in particular the Ruffini receptors and interstitial receptors. These sensors send signals to the spinal cord, which in turn changes the muscle tension or the dilation of the blood vessels. The fascia and the signals it sends to the nervous system and the brain are therefore driving factors behind these phenomena that physical therapists and physicians have long been aware of, but of which they knew very little regarding the specific origin and mode of action (Chapter 4, physiotherapy).

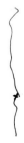

Waterman fights against this loss and his illness: he wants to train his movements consciously—and it works, albeit with great effort. Every movement has to be controlled by him deliberately, rather than instinctively.

This is all about vision. When Ian is in a lit room and the light is switched off, he falls to the ground, because he sees nothing and his conscious control fails: the body has no organ for internal movement control. I was able to meet him in person at a scientific investigation, and was incredibly impressed by his battle against the sensory motion blindness. Walking and moving are for Ian a daily marathon—for a healthy person these actions generally happen unconsciously. He is also the only man of all known cases who has managed to walk again independently—truly a masterstroke.

The BBC has published documentation about Ian Waterman's history. It is still available on the web under the title "The Man Who Lost His Body".

The Importance of Fascia

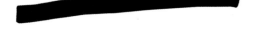

- Muscles cannot work or keep their shape without their fascial envelopes—they would simply flow apart like viscous syrup.

- The number of sensors in the fascia exceeds by far the number of sensors of the muscles.

- The fascia reports information about movement, position, tension, pressure, and pain to the somatic central nervous system and to the autonomic nervous system.

- The fascia is our largest sensory organ by area—even larger than the skin.

- The bodywide fascia net is the crucial organ for body perception.

THE SCIENCE OF FASCIA

All the findings that have been accumulated by various fascia researchers throughout the world are as yet not absolutely clear in terms of their scope. One thing for certain is that they have changed the opinion of physicians concerning many disease patterns. They also present completely new aspects with regard to anatomy, exercise science, regulation of body functions, phenomena such as scarring and wound healing, and even mental health and brain function.

Of course, modern fascia researchers did not start from the very beginning. In the 19th century, evidence of the performance of the connective tissue was available, and pioneers have since made some groundbreaking discoveries. Some of the people involved were established histologists, such as Alfred Pischinger; others were clinical scientists, such as the biochemist Ida P. Rolf. However, there were also physiotherapists, such as Elisabeth Dicke, or autodidacts with very little formal medical training, such as Andrew Taylor Still, the founder of osteopathy. They all stressed the importance of connective tissue, physical movement, and manual therapy—aspects which we can scientifically investigate today.

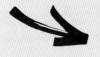

Alfred Pischinger and
His System of Basic Regulation

Alfred Pischinger (1899–1983) was an Austrian histologist and embryologist, who taught as a professor of medicine at the University of Graz and later in Vienna, where he also carried out medical research.

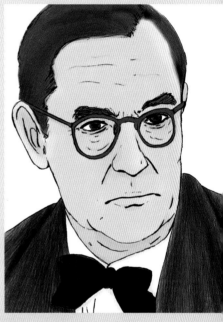

Alfred Pischinger pictured the human body as a self-regulating and networked system, in which information about different subsystems is passed on and processed. In his view the connective tissue had a key role as an intermediary that had effects on vital basic functions, such as blood pressure and immune defense; he named this role *ground regulation*. He described the treatment as *holistic* because it takes into account the interconnected nature of the organism.

His image of cells and their metabolism was that of a friendly environment, which the cell needs like a unicellular organism needs seawater. Via this milieu the cell obtains nutrients, disposes of metabolites, and exchanges signals. The way the cell communicates with its environment is a two-way relationship. All the surrounded cells are dependent on this environment—the matrix.

As early as 1933 Austrian Pischinger became a member of the Nazi party. He was a supporting member of the SS, and later, while at the University of Graz, he became a leading member of a group of Nazi doctors who dealt with eugenics. This Nazi past unfortunately raises a shadow over his otherwise tremendously valuable accomplishments. After the war and a denazification, Pischinger became a professor in Vienna, where he was highly honored for his physiological research. He died there in 1983.

From Body Therapist to Researcher

My personal interest in fascia was first stimulated by practical work: since the 1980s I have had a Rolfing practice in Munich, which was so interesting that I gave up my clinical practice as a psychologist. Physically working with the human body was so much more exciting to me. In 1988 I began to occupy myself more with the theories behind Rolfing. That said, I also began to question those theories. Some dogmas seemed doubtful, and some of the explanations of our pioneer Ida Rolf no longer satisfied me as such. According to the Rolf doctrine, the fascia are solid collagenous material that create a body frame which we therapists should form and deform with our hands like putty or chewing gum—and this on a

As a Rolfer, I experienced fascia work for the first time.

sustainable basis. I have not experienced that during my work—but I knew that I, as a therapist, certainly triggered something: the tissue, the muscles, and the posture of my patients literally changed in my hands. This occurred not only because of strong pressure, but often also because of the minute and gentle melting movements required by Rolfing therapy.

But there had to be other mechanisms. Further explanations were thrown into the mix, but they too were unsatisfactory: for example, energy flow, meridians, and blockages—interpretations that feature in the usual fashionable esoteric kit. I wanted to look at the other point of view—the scientific aspect. Ida Rolf herself was a biochemist, and in my psychology studies in Heidelberg I had learned something about the basic principles of scientific thinking and serious scientific research— about medical and psychological methods in statistics, the biological basis, the nervous system and the main body functions. I thought that if we Rolfers and manual therapists were successful, then this success would also be reflected in a modern world view and there would be traceable, measurable effects on the body.

In 2002, after a decade of teaching at the Rolf Institute I treated myself to a year off, to find answers to some nagging scientific questions. As a Rolfer I gained my first experience with fascia work. I obtained study material from physiologists and

Elisabeth Dicke and
Connective Tissue Massage

Elisabeth Dicke (1884–1952) was a physiotherapist, and following her training in the 1920s, she ran a private practice in Wuppertal Barmen. In 1929 she suffered circulatory problems and leg pain, as well as renal colic and an inflammatory swelling of the liver. She also had a firm swelling in the subcutaneous tissue of the abdomen. She healed herself through self-massage, even to a certain extent in the more distant locations of her body, such as the back and pelvis. According to her own information, this enabled her to remedy the pain.

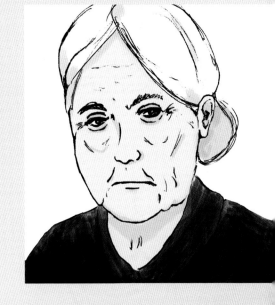

In 1938 Elisabeth Dicke and Hede Teirich-Leube developed their method of connective tissue massage. Both women were physiotherapists and assumed that the connective tissue was an organ with a connection to the somatic and autonomic nervous systems. Their assumption was supported by neurological findings of sensitive skin areas that the British neurologist Henry Head had described. Their new massage technique stimulated these zones, leading to basic responses, such as relaxation, reduced blood pressure, and a slowing of the pulse. The treatment apparently also had an impact on the internal organs, and pain was alleviated.

Unfortunately, Elisabeth Dicke did not live long enough to see the success of their method: after her death the connective tissue massage was medically approved and validated neurologically and physiologically. In 1968 Hede Teirich-Leube received the Order of Merit for her services. She died in 1979.

Ida Rolf, Founder of Rolfing and Structural Integration

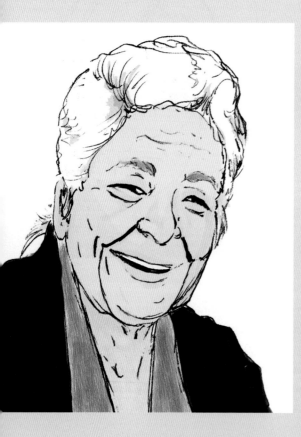

Ida P. Rolf (1896–1979) studied biochemistry, and in 1920 she was one of the first women in the United States to receive her doctorate in this subject. She worked as a researcher at the Rockefeller Institute, examining infectious diseases and threats to public health. The institute became a center for clinical studies. She carried out intensive work on chemistry and medical mathematics, but also on alternative therapies, including chiropractic, osteopathy, and homeopathy.

Performing treatment tests on family members and friends, Ida Rolf developed her manual therapy and structural integration, which was later called *Rolfing*. When someone experiences pain, poor posture, and tension, this type of therapy considers the main cause to be in the connective tissue rather than in the muscles and bones. Ida Rolf was convinced that the connective tissue and the structural alignment of the whole body can be influenced by manual therapy.

She largely based her therapy on mechanical factors, because she knew that the connective tissue was a collageneous and a malleable material; she therefore wanted to influence the tissue mainly through physical input, such as pressure and traction. As early as 1971 she considered the body to be a network of fascia. But she also believed in the psychological effects of manual stimulation: after a successful Rolfing series she expected that not only should a faulty posture be corrected, but also anxiety, low self-esteem, and depression should be attenuated.

Ida P. Rolf is now considered one of the pioneers of fascia treatment—the Rolfing method has now spread worldwide. Researchers and therapists who work in this field include leading fascia experts, such as the rehabilitation physicians Thomas Findley and Thomas Myers, who developed the system of myofascial meridians.

doctors on the subject of connective tissue and attended numerous congresses. With amazement I read Professor Jochen Staubesand's work in 1996—he showed that the fascia contains cells which are able to contract. He believed that these were smooth muscle cells, and he conjectured that these very cells might be controlled by the autonomic nervous system. That fascinated me, and I began to call universities and look for researchers who were willing to talk to me—a mere practitioner of alternative Rolfing therapy. That was not easy. Some just laughed at me or responded neither to my phone messages nor to my repeated polite letters. Finally, I met Professor Frank Lehmann-Horn at the University of Ulm, a renowned neurophysiologist who researched rare muscle diseases; he was an expert. He regarded the muscles and fascia as a unit when it comes to body motion, and was precisely the teacher and mentor I was looking for. He accepted my proposal to begin a program of experimental research with him; that became the basis of my doctorate in human biology.

When we finally succeeded in proving in the laboratory at Ulm that fascia reacts to certain chemical messengers and is populated by muscle-like cells, which allows it to actively contract, a new path was mapped out for me. I wanted to continue to work hands-on as a therapist—but I wanted to connect with other scientific fascia researchers and gain as much insight into the fascia as possible. Let me mention here just a few examples— findings which are important corner pieces of the big puzzle for fascia researchers.

▦ Revolutionary Discoveries

I have been working at the University of Ulm since 2003, and now direct a department there called 'Fascia Research Group'. Recent scientific fascia research has emerged from many areas of medicine—histology, physiology, anatomy, and neurology. Moreover, since the development of new imaging and molecular techniques, the exploration of the fascia has of course gone much deeper than it did at the beginning of the 20th century.

I will mention only a few findings and discoveries by colleagues in recent years:

- The fascia of the lower back in humans is densely populated with specialized pain receptors and is the location in which back pain frequently starts to develop, as shown by the pain researcher Siegfried Mense in Heidelberg.

- Fascia forms a body-wide signaling network, as described by the neurophysiologist and Harvard professor of complementary therapies Helene Langevin in Vermont (USA). A researcher also in acupuncture, yoga, and other methods, she has moreover been able to prove a correlation of particular fascial densification lines with the so-called meridians in the Chinese therapy method of acupuncture. The success of acupuncture can partly be explained by its effect on the fascia and its provable neurobiological effects. Langevin has contributed new insights in yoga and massage. (More details can be found in Chapter 4 on physiotherapy.)

- Scar-like adhesions in the fascia can be influenced by gentle massage and significantly improve, as the physiotherapist Susan Chapelle and the physiologist Geoffrey Bove have shown in animal studies. The animals concerned had scars and fascial adhesions in the abdomen; they were divided into different groups, and one group was gently massaged every day with techniques similar to Rolfing. These animals were later found to have less intra-abdominal adhesions than those which were not massaged.

- Fascia can contract independently from muscles and can react to messenger substances that are associated with emotional stress—a

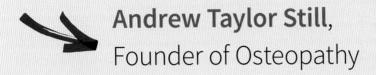

Andrew Taylor Still,
Founder of Osteopathy

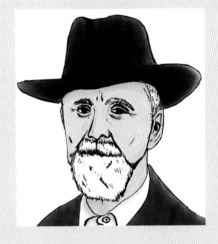

Andrew Taylor Still (1828–1917) was a field physician and natural healer in the United States who had no formal medical training. He learned the basic medical principles from his father (who himself was a doctor), and took a few courses at various institutes. He was not a graduate of a regular course of study. In his country doctor's office he worked mostly using naturopathic methods—such as cupping, bloodletting, leeching, and dieting—but he was also sympathetic to esoteric influences, such as skull science, mesmerism, and spiritualism.

In 1870 Andrew Taylor Still turned to manual methods and undertook anatomical studies. He discovered that treatments with his hands helped patients. In certain diseases, he found hard spots in the muscles or in the skin, which could be influenced by pressure and massage, and partly by merely laying his hands on the patient's body. This is how he developed the principles of his teaching about the healing powers of the organism, which had to be triggered by touch, as well as about the fundamental importance of exercise for the human body.

In 1892 he and his family founded a school in Kansas for the treatment that Still himself called *osteopathy*.

As one of the very first innovators, Still emphasized that fascia is supplied by nerves and is to be regarded as a sensory organ. Some of his intuitive insights into the fascia as a member of the body-wide regulation system and the autonomic nervous system have now been confirmed by physiologists.

result from our work in the Fascia Research Laboratory at the University of Ulm. This phenomenon is due to specific types of connective tissue cells, namely *myofibroblasts*, which are very frequently found in the lumbar fascia. In wound healing these cells are responsible for the wound closure and scar formation. There are specialized devices in the matrix regulation of soft connective tissues with a very strong contractile force. Myofibroblasts and their contraction of the fascia may also be one reason why musculoskeletal pain is often found to accompany chronic emotional stress.

When muscles contract, their force transmission to the joints is often dramatically altered by the surrounding fascial tissues. This was recently demonstrated by the biomechanics and movement researcher Peter Huijing. There are significant differences from individual to individual concerning this feature. Huijing's research on spastic paralyzed children and the involvement of the fascia has been recognized with international awards.

New results from all corners of the world are added daily to this list. Above all there are also many additional practical therapies, whether they be on the diagnosis side (for example, using a new ultrasound machine, which can show images of soft tissues, such as fascia), or on the treatment side (for example, patients with lower back pain, who could not be helped either by strength training or even by painkillers). It may sound hard to believe, but it is impossible to predict what the future has to offer.

Fascia promises to provide an explanation for many cases of low back pain, which is the number one complaint and one of the most costly. The number of interoceptors in the fascia exceeds by far the number of mechanoreceptors (movement, position, pressure, etc.). This highlights the great importance of these signals for the state and activity of the organs in the body.

Our "gut feeling," that is the internal perception of bodily functions and organ activities, seems to depend especially on the fascia, the connective tissue of the viscera. The signals from the fascia go to the brain—and in there to the so-called *island area* (insula) of the cerebrum. Incidentally, this is the region with which brain researchers connect the sense of self and our emotional state. In this way, what we call *consciousness* could be dependent on body sensation and on the perception and processing of numerous signals from our fascia.

Mental illnesses—such as depression, anxiety disorders, and others—are today explained by disorders of interception, for which neurophysiological signals from the interceptors in the fascia are responsible.

The human subcutaneous connective tissue has a special sensory system for affective touch, which are responsive to gentle skin contact, stroking, and social touch. This system is also connected to the brain, again to the insula, the center for consciousness, self-awareness, empathy, emotions, and social skills.

Have I now raved enough about the paramount importance of fascia? As you can tell, I am fascinated by this subject. This fascination is also due to the many dedicated and inspiring colleagues around the world who in recent years have exchanged their findings and who are working together on the new image of a body-wide interconnected fibrous network, called fascia. The spirit of discovery and excitement that characterizes this field is indeed contagious—and I admit that makes me happy. In the year 2000 or so when I tried to make contact with researchers and scientists in this field, I stood in front of many closed doors and had to wait a long, long time to get an appointment or a meeting, if ever. Today, many of the same researchers call on me and my fascia researcher colleagues for knowledge and advice.

A cross section through the skin, showing the fascial layers—superficial and deep fascia.

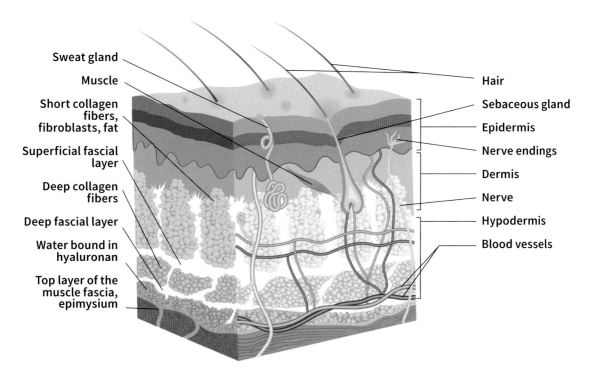

- Sweat gland
- Muscle
- Short collagen fibers, fibroblasts, fat
- Superficial fascial layer
- Deep collagen fibers
- Deep fascial layer
- Water bound in hyaluronan
- Top layer of the muscle fascia, epimysium
- Hair
- Sebaceous gland
- Epidermis
- Nerve endings
- Dermis
- Nerve
- Hypodermis
- Blood vessels

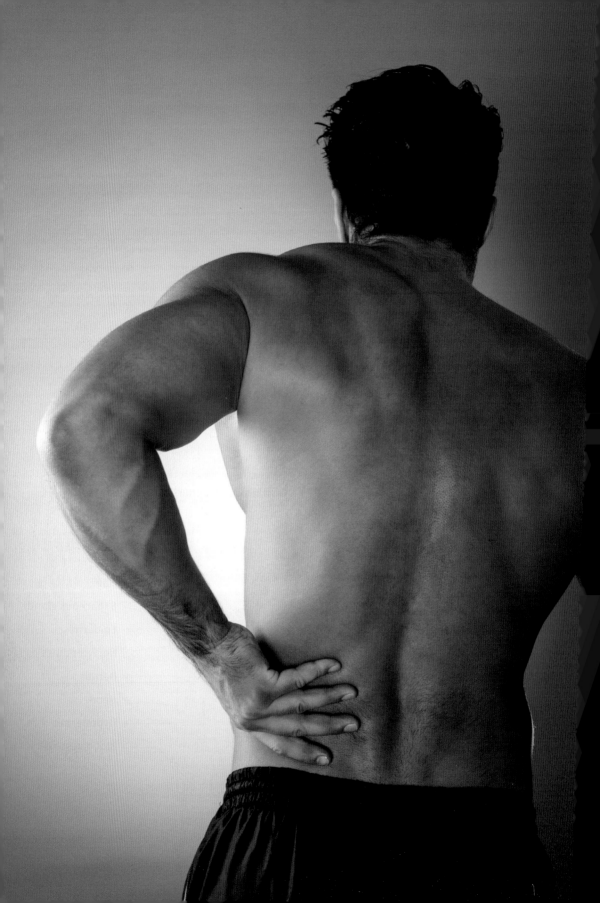

Backache: A Common Illness and New Perspectives

The causes of chronic back pain, now a common disease and one of the most common causes of disability and early retirement, have not as yet been adequately explained. The usual suspects are intervertebral discs, vertebrae, nerves, or weak and incorrectly exercised muscles. Many disc and vertebral operations do not lead to a permanent improvement. Conversely, there are many people with visible intervertebral disc and vertebral damage who are completely healthy and pain-free. Muscle training does not always help—even well-trained athletes can suffer from back pain.

Fascia research now sheds new light on the problem. First, we have learned that fascia is densely populated with pain sensors, especially in the back. We then saw that because the fascia possesses contractile cells, it contracts under the influence of certain substances. Studies carried out on male patients with back pain have shown that their lumbar fascia, which covers a large area, is clearly thickened in the lower back region; and it does not slide as freely as it does in healthy persons. Often this leads to a characteristic gait. All this suggests that disorders or problems in the back fascia contribute to pain, or that these pathologies might even originate there. Small injuries or tearing in the fascia caused by irregular and one-sided strain may play an important role. Such micro-injuries to the fascia could cause inflammation, as well as corrupted signaling about joint position, which are then transmitted from the fascia to the muscles. The subsequent muscular dysfunction causes further cramping; both of these together could lead to chronic back pain. This has given rise to a worldwide discussion among researchers about the participation of the fascia in the creation of soft tissue pain.

The pain is deep down in the back. Reason unknown.
Could the solution to the mystery be in the fascia?

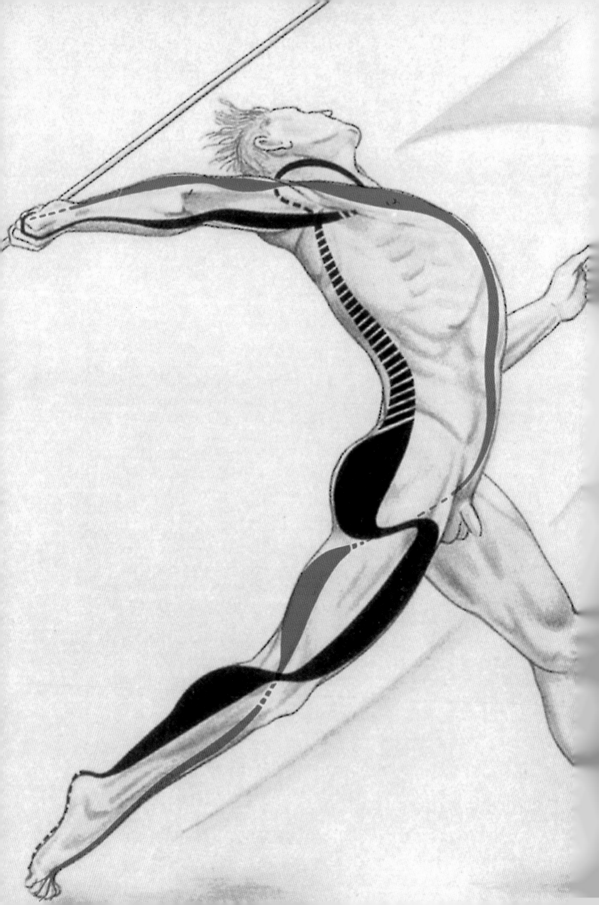

CHAPTER 2

Principles of Fascia Training

Training is definitely a question of fashion: there have been popular trends such as stretching and aerobics or Callanetics, and Asian martial arts styles along with yoga and Pilates. We have training with equipment and without, with a partner or alone, indoors, outdoors, with instructions, with music, with exercises to follow on DVD, and with weekly schedules and diet programs. The main theme of all training, however, is movement.

Ultimately, scientific knowledge should be able to help in improving or refreshing training programs, which has indeed happened in recent years as a result of fascia research. Incorporating knowledge about the functionality of fascia can influence previous training methods and normal exercising.

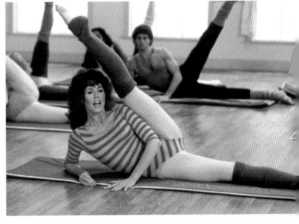

A trend from the 1980s: Jane Fonda and fitness for women.

You do not have to discard or replace everything that you are used to, however, because much can be easily integrated into existing programs.

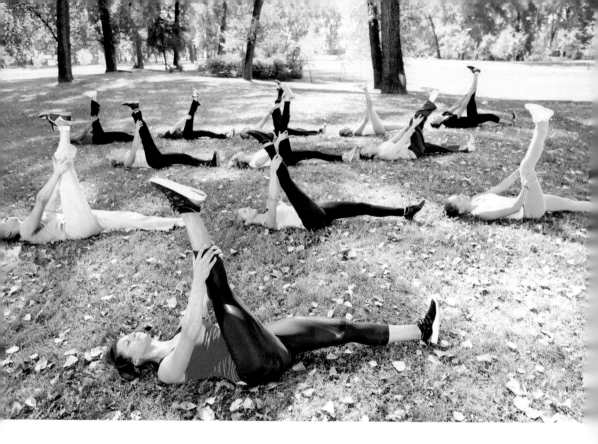

Stretching before exercise should protect against injuries – in my opinion.

The new fascia exercises merely widen the spectrum—they do not radically change it. If you are clear about the role of fascia in motion, you can also improve your performance using a program that you already follow. Even if you are not currently following a training regime, you can learn about fascia awareness and set up easy exercises; this will give you a wonderful introduction to healthy exercise.

Fascia training therefore does not replace any previous training programs; it complements and enriches them by means of a component that has generally been missing. In other words, it simply completes the picture. Fascia training offers to present an additional pillar to the current emphasis on muscular, cardiovascular, and coordination training—it adds the finishing touch to your personal training program. This applies to athletes at all levels—but not just to athletes.

HEALTHY MOVEMENT IN EVERYDAY LIFE

Our goal is not limited to achieving a better athletic performance. The fascia workout has enormous importance for everyday movement, as well as for prevention and rehabilitation in the case of injury. Healthy exercise in everyday life is particularly close to my heart.

I believe that life in the modern world limits us in our natural motion: we no longer move as much and as diversely as our ancestral forefathers, whose bodies we inherited, used to move. Our daily movement repertoire is no longer natural for our species (for example, office work requires us to sit in an unnatural, cramped position with continuous long hours of immobility). Even during walking and running, we are hampered by poor-quality equipment on our feet—here I mean shoes. You will learn more about the topics of gait and feet in this chapter; in a later section you will find out even more, because fascia research brings to light a new impetus.

Musculoskeletal pain is so widespread that some sceptics say: "A person over 40 years of age who wakes up in the morning without pain is probably deceased." As we already know, frequent disturbances in the fascia probably cause many of these pain problems and diseases—and that is precisely the reason why the fascia system in our body should always be well maintained. This applies particularly to people who have to sit a lot. The reason is—the fascia needs specific movement in order to stay healthy.

Especially in the middle of our lives, it becomes increasingly important for the fascia to be "fit." The contorted body shape—

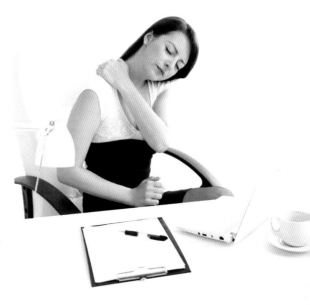

At times, we may suffer from pain in the neck and shoulder due to incorrect working positions.

the typical senior profile of a hunched torso and forward-bent shoulders—is to a large extent a result of aging of the fascia. The dreaded stiffness that comes with age arises from the fact that the connective tissue becomes clotted and fibrotic with advancing years because of a lack of training. The problem is not just a cosmetic one: even falls and injuries and musculoskeletal pain are related to declining mobility.

If the fascia is fit and in good condition, a youthful, toned body shape and an elastic mobility can be maintained for a long time. So if you want to stay young, or to be young again, you will do well to strengthen this "web of life." Living bodies function according to the "use it or lose it!" principle;

in particular, the bones, muscles, tendons, and fascia are constantly being assembled and disassembled, in order to better adapt to the movements imposed on them.

What we do not need or ordinarily require, the body regards as unwanted ballast and therefore tries to reduce it in order to save energy. Conversely, the muscles and fasciae we do need and train on a regular basis remain intact.

The hunched posture of older people has its origin in the state of the fascia.

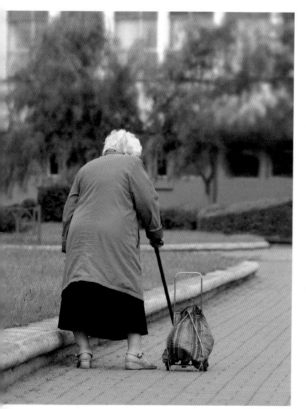

In old age we can specifically train so as to influence the number and interconnections of neurons in our brain in order to increase both bone and muscle mass. This also applies to the quality of our fascia.

WHAT YOU SHOULD KNOW BEFORE YOU TRAIN

In this chapter we will take a closer look at the function of the fascia specifically in the human musculoskeletal system, to understand which tasks need to be performed by the muscles and the interaction of these muscles with the fascia. We also consider the importance of fascial tissue not only for mobility and joints, but also for the body shape. I present to you a new concept of the body which is not based upon rigid, mechanically connected bones, but rather consists of a dynamic network, composed of long and elastic fascial connections. At the end of this chapter there is a self-test, which you can use to determine your natural type of connective tissue. All this is important for selecting the exercises that you will get to know later and will hopefully try out.

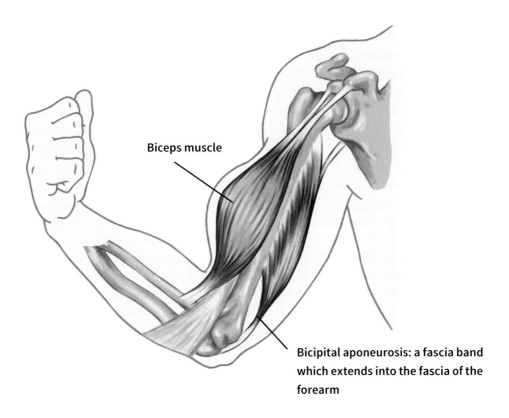

Biceps muscle

Bicipital aponeurosis: a fascia band which extends into the fascia of the forearm

The biceps muscle is attached to the shoulder and forearm bones by tendons, which give tension to the bone. A broad fascial band transmits additional forces below the elbow.

If they so wish, impatient readers can skip ahead and go directly to the exercises, which are presented in Chapter 3, along with pictures and descriptions. However, to be honest I would advise you to read the following sections on the importance of fascia for human movement and to then perform the self-test. This knowledge will then help you in understanding the exercises, and will motivate you to do them!

HOW MUSCLE AND FASCIA COOPERATE

As we saw in Chapter 2, muscle and fascia form a common structure. But the fascia also has distinct functions relating to movement, to structure and posture of the body, and also to body shape.

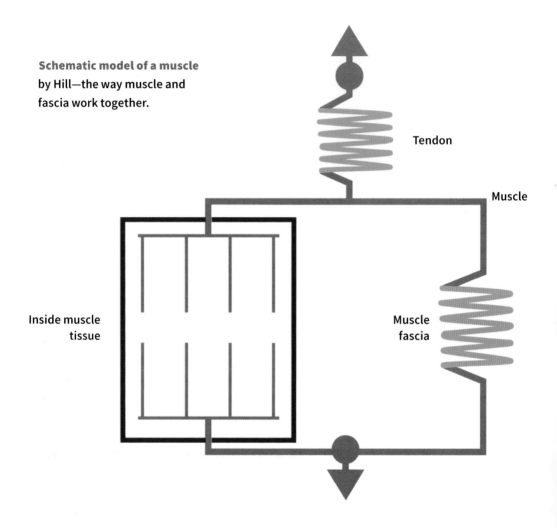

Schematic model of a muscle by Hill—the way muscle and fascia work together.

Tendon

Muscle

Inside muscle tissue

Muscle fascia

We will begin with the function of the fascia in and around the muscles themselves, where—from a purely anatomical standpoint—it is described as envelopes around fibers and fiber bundles, as well as around the entire muscle. But what exactly does the fascia do here?

We learned in Chapter 1 that each individual fiber of a muscle is wrapped in fascia. The task these fascia cases fulfill with regard to power transmission is related to the mechanics of the muscle and to the complete movement. To enable the limbs to move, the muscles need a connection to the bones. This connection is provided by sinews, or tendons, of collagenous fibers that are fused with the periosteum, or specific attachment points on the bones. Tendons can be seen as tight fascia composed of densely packed and very strong collagen fibers.

The transition between bone and tendon is a smooth continuation: from bone to cartilage, and then to tendon, which then attaches to muscle. There are also specialized connective tissue cells between tendon and muscle; this creates a continuum of fascial tissue that bears the mechanical strength of the muscle.

The fact that a large portion of the force of the muscle reaches the tendon, and that this tension passes to the bone at all, occurs thanks to the performance of the fascial envelopes in and around the muscle. The role these fascial containers play is that of a mediator of force.

Fascia gains tension from the contraction of many muscle fibers and passes it on, from the endomysium to the perimysium and epimysium, and then to the tendon, where the forces finally reach the bone. The effect of muscle strength is thus based specifically on the cooperation of muscle and fascia. Biomechanical engineers picture this using the image of a feather.

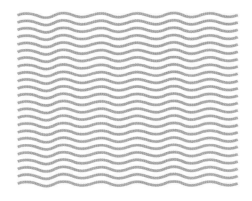

The regular 'waves' of healthy fascia.

must therefore be able change its shape in response to mechanical tension, and when the tension is released, it must return to its original form. We already know from Chapter 1 that fascia is made of elastic material, primarily collagen. It is a characteristic of elastic material that the energy applied to it—the tension—is stored as energy and then released again.

The force of the impact and the rebound are linked in a manner which is dictated by the material. Elastic material with a high capacity to store energy bounces back sharply, as in the case of a metal spring or a rubber band; the same applies to the fascia which encases the muscles and tendons.

■ **Springiness as a Measure of the Quality of Fascia**

Elastic springiness is a very important factor and plays a central role in the ability of the fascia to move. But the ability of a structure to spring and bounce means that something within it has to be elastic; the material

In addition, the tissue of muscle fascia is arranged in regular waves. This is called 'crimping'. This wavy alignment increases the ability to store energy. The structure has the appearance of wavy hair; the stronger

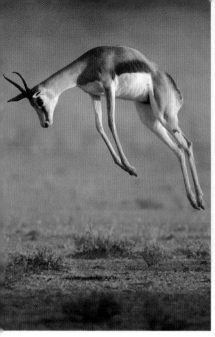
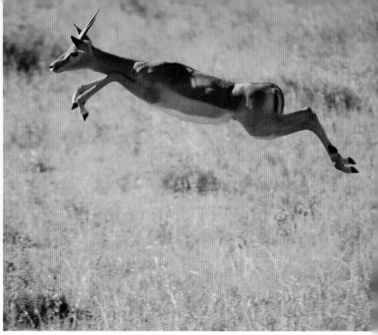

Championship high jump and long jump: gazelles and antelopes.

the waves are, the more elastic rebound capacity the fascia will have. With age, this corrugation gradually decreases—but with the right training, it can be restored.

Resilience and the ability to store and release elastic energy are essential features of the fascia and tendons. Both of these properties allow elegant dynamic movements, as biomechanical engineers have found from observations of antelopes and kangaroos. These animals can jump incredibly high and long: small antelopes manage to jump to a height of 3 m and a distance of 10 m, whereas red kangaroos can jump more than 13 m, which is further than any other animal. The red kangaroo can also run as fast as a racehorse—up to 60 km per hour.

This extraordinary performance, however, can only be explained to a minor degree

by their muscle strength. Antelopes and gazelles are delicate creatures and do not have large muscle masses, but their graceful limbs do have long tendons. The long hind legs of kangaroos are remarkable, and they have very strong Achilles tendons with a very high elastic storage ability. Indeed, the combination of the elastic tendons

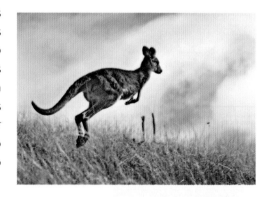

A kangaroo jumping: the long hind legs bounce off the ground.

56

and the long legs of both kangaroos and antelopes is responsible for their amazing performance. The huge leaps that these animals can make are due to the ingenious mechanism of the fascia.

▥ The Catapult Effect

How the spring effect works can be explained biomechanically by a comparison to the mechanism of a catapult; this implement hurls something forward as a result of it being placed under mechanical strain. When this tension is suddenly discharged, the stored energy is transformed into kinetic energy, and the load is propelled forward. Another very simple example is a rubber band which is stretched and then quickly released. In the case of a rubber ball falling to the ground, the impact exerts pressure on the rubber, which then deforms and charges up with energy; it then snaps back to its original shape—and rises off the ground again.

Throwing with tensile energy: the catapult.

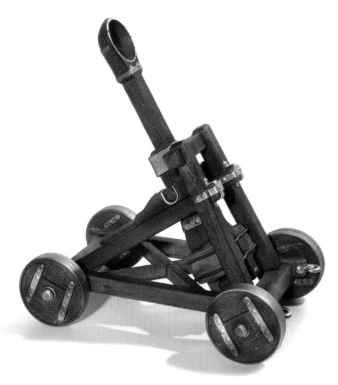

The rebound effect therefore makes it possible to move around with a minimum of muscle strength. The muscles also produce a triggering contraction, which puts tension on the tendons. After the first jump, all subsequent jumps rely mainly on gravity and individual weight. When the body bounces back onto the floor, the ankle and the Achilles tendon compress and reload with energy. The combined energy then discharges, and the rebound may have an acceleration that exceeds the speed of highly trained muscles. Animals such as gazelles, antelopes, and kangaroos jump in a very energy-efficient way, mainly because their tendons are repeatedly absorbing and releasing mechanical force.

The situation is different when jumping from a standing position, such as a frog leaping suddenly into the air like a rocket. Or imagine, for example, a cat jumping from the ground up onto a high table. The cat crouches down and quickly stretches the muscles that act on its long tendons. Before the cat jumps, these muscles twitch as quickly as possible, which puts strain on the tendons; and finally the tendons releases this tension with a much faster speed than the original muscular contraction.

This rebound effect of the tendons and fascia is a universal biomechanical principle in rapidly moving animals—and in humans too. Our hopping and jumping, as well as running and walking, benefit especially from this catapult effect. Biomechanical engineers have discovered that the ability of fascia to store mechanical energy is very similar between humans and gazelles.

The capacity of our tendons to store energy surpasses that of all other primates: humans are the only primate with those gazelle-like running and jumping tendons. Homo sapiens has evolved this elastic storage capacity of the fascia in our legs to a much greater degree than its climbing relatives.

■ Our Best Discipline: Walking

Humans are known to be able to develop an impressive endurance in walking. We can hike for hours with almost no fatigue; this comes as no surprise, as researchers have discovered. Thanks to the catapult mechanism, walking requires only very little muscular energy. This miracle of movement happens because of a chain of fascia, ranging from the large plantar fascia in our feet to the Achilles tendon on the heel, then via a fascial muscle chain all the way up to our back. Fascia and muscles work together in a larger functional unit, which extends longer than the two muscular attachment points to the skeleton.

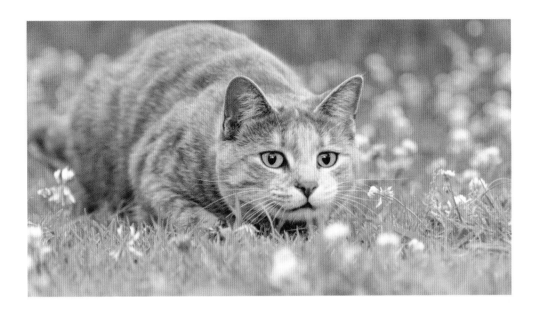

Ready to jump: the cat crouches, tenses its muscles and tendons, and then boosts its jump through tension.

The fact that we can walk so effectively is attributable to one of the longer fascia chains that run through the body—in this case, along our back. It stretches over the feet and legs, along with the Achilles tendon at the rear, to the large lumbar fascia, and then further up to the neck and on to the scalp on our head. Since this chain of fascia can store a lot of energy and subsequently release it with hardly any muscular intervention, the human gait is very efficient and enduring.

We should therefore train our fascia and keep it fit, in order to maintain and improve its elasticity and energy storage capacity. Only those tendons and fascia that are in good shape and have the right structure can efficiently store energy and release it dynamically.

FASCIAL CHAINS AND THE ENERGY NETWORK

The overarching fascia mechanics, as I have described with reference to walking and the back fascia line, influences the types of exercise that are beneficial. When walking around there is far more fascia involved than just that in our feet—this is characteristic of the fascia in the body as a whole. It runs over the joints and individual limbs, and courses through the body like a network. There are long chains of muscle fascia units that run like long elastic slings through the body and are responsible for posture, stability, and efficient, fluid movement.

These long connections between muscles and fasciae had been neglected in sports and medicine for a very long time. However, they have received increasing interest during recent years. A particularly plausible and detailed model for this system was described by my Rolfing colleague Thomas W. Myers, who developed it in the 1990s. Myers is a Rolfing practitioner and was an anatomy instructor at the Ida Rolf Institute; he was also trained in the Feldenkrais method and has a deep understanding of many therapeutic bodywork modalities. His system of long myofascial chains in the body, which was mostly derived from practical work, has now been reconfirmed in many aspects by anatomical researchers.

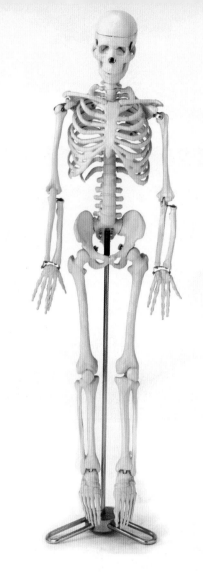

A skeleton cannot stand upright on its own—it always needs a prop, as this model shows.

▥ The Skeleton Is Not Scaffolding

Myers' model goes along with the following premises: it is not so much the bones that keep the body upright and supported, but this function is essentially fulfilled by the fascia. You can see that just from the fact that a skeleton cannot stand erect unaided; without support it would simply fall apart. The skeleton therefore cannot serve well as a scaffolding, which provides stability for adjacent parts.

Sailboat Principle: The Spine

For several years medical and orthopedic practitioners have used the image of a sailboat with mast, shrouds, and rigging to describe the static conditions in the spine. Such a mast does not carry much load by itself, but serves as a stable element within a larger tensile bracing system. Many ropes reinforce this system and provide stability. The mast does not carry weight like a column—similarly to our back. A healthy human spine is bendable and is responsive to tensional forces from external myofascial chains.

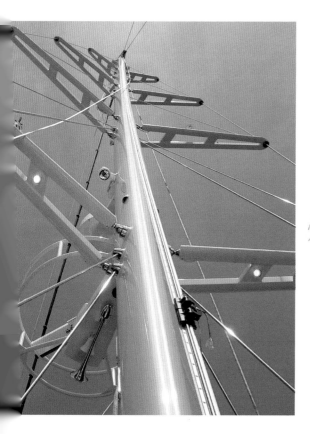

Mast of a sailboat.

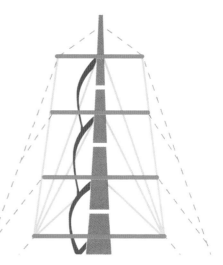

The sailboat principle of the spine, medically speaking, is that in the back there are ligaments and muscles which are under tension, keeping the spine erect. In the middle lies the intrinsic back musculature; all other structures extend transversely, accommodating various external muscles.

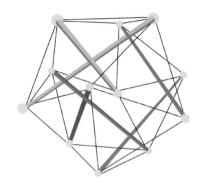

A tensegrity model: the tension provides a system with both stability and dynamics.

What keeps the body upright is a dynamic network of fascia and muscles maintained in a state of tension. We know, for instance, that remaining upright requires constant slight adjustments in muscle tension and in order to stay in balance. If we do not do this, we fall to the ground; when we sleep deeply we normally cannot stand upright because muscle tonicity ceases to function. The muscle tension in turn is conveyed through the fascia, which provides a body-wide supporting network.

▤ The Tensegrity Model

Such tensional networks are increasingly imitated in modern architecture. They are called *tensegrity* models; the neologism "tensegrity" is composed of the words "tension" and "integrity." Structures with that name were developed in the mid-20th century by American artists and architects. They tend to have the following characteristics:

- They consist of sturdy and elastic elements.

- The elastic elements are under constant tension.

- The sturdy elements are connected to each other only by the elastic elements.

- The sturdy elements do not transmit compression directly to each other.

- All elastic elements are connected with each other and thus provide a tensional network throughout the whole system.

Fascia researchers assume that the construction of a healthy human body contains many similarities with such a tensegrity system: the long fascial muscle chains form a network of continuous tension in which the organs and bones are elastically suspended.

This system is very sensitive to movement—it is dynamic. If we activate a muscle in one place, a reaction somewhere else in the body is transmitted through the long myofascial chains to which it is connected. Muscles do not work well by themselves; they are always linked together in the body's fascial network. This way of thinking goes beyond the classical anatomy approach of individually localized muscles: it identifies larger functional fascia units in the body.

▥ A New Concept of the Body

This new concept of the body has some important consequences, including the current understanding of bones and joints. In fact, almost nowhere in the body do bones directly touch each other. Almost always they are flexibly interconnected by connective tissue—cartilage, capsules, ligaments, and tendons. If one thinks in this way, then one's concept of the spine also changes. The spine is not a central pillar like that in an ancient temple; it is instead one of 33 vertebrae that are aligned like many pieces of cork connected by an elastic rope. The backbone therefore is not a continuous bone, like the femur, but consists of an alignment of numerous flexible joints, which are held together by bands and a whole system of fascia and small muscles.

Fascia researchers now re-examine all issues of body posture and upright walking in terms of the dynamic network that runs throughout the body, especially in the back. For example one of the topics of our research group at Ulm University is to investigate the interactions between human gait, the elastic storage capacity of healthy lumbodorsal fascia and a potential link with the development or prevention of low back pain.

▥ The Fascial Chains of the Body

Our body is therefore made up of a whole network of different tensile elements, within which some longer myofascial chains can now be identified. In our opinion these myofascial chains play a special role in smooth and elegant movement coordination; they therefore need to be stimulated and emphasized during exercising, so that coordination and proper function is trained throughout these chains. Isolated exercises for individual muscle groups, as in normal strength training, are not adequate for this purpose. From our fascial perspective, the remote connections across the body are important, and we want to specifically activate the training of these. For this you need to be aware of the most important fascial chains of the body:

- Superficial back line

- Superficial front line

- Two lateral lines

- Spiral line

These long chains extend over the length of the body, across several specific parts, and along the limbs; they have both static and dynamic functions, as accurately described by Thomas Myers. In this book their discussion will be confined to the most significant points.

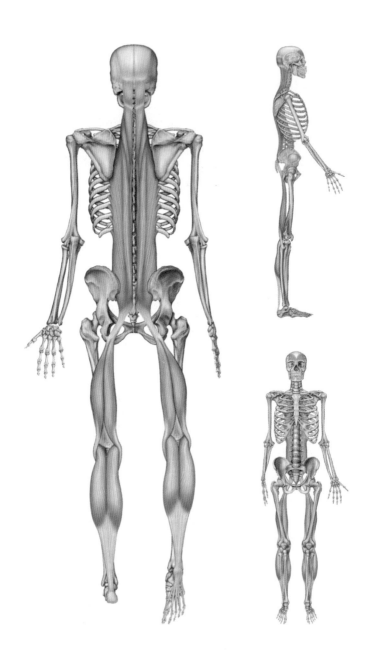

● 1. Superficial Back Line

The superficial back line runs from the feet (plantar fascia) to the back, neck, and head, up to the eyebrows. It supports and protects the back and is responsible for upright posture and for extending the torso upward and backward.

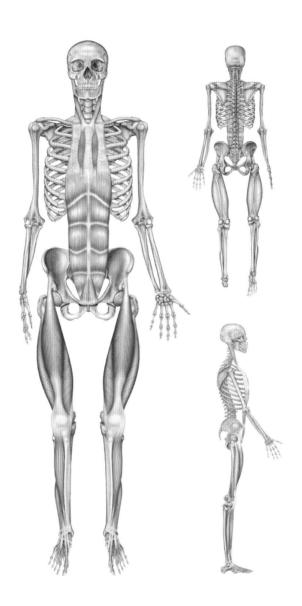

● 2. Superficial Front Line

The superficial front line runs from the toes to the pelvis, then up the belly to the neck and head. Although it consists of two parts, in an upright body position it acts as a single link from top to bottom.

Its function is to stabilize the upper body posture; it also allows movements and bending, as well as lifting and lowering of the upper body.

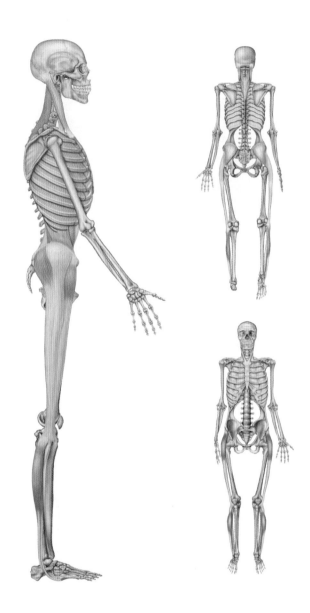

● **3. Lateral Lines**

The lateral lines run along each side of the body and enclose both outer sides. They begin on the outside of the foot, skirt around the outside of the ankle, pass further upward, and then, like a basket, weave up the sides of the body to the head. These lines ensure balance between the front and back lines, and connect our torso and legs, so that they do not give way suddenly. They are also involved in side bending of the body, and also curb excessive bending and rotation.

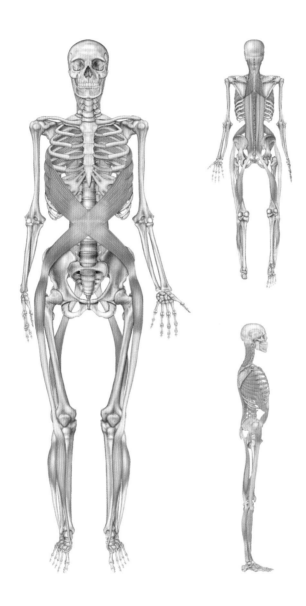

● 4. Spiral Line

The spiral line winds around the body, allows rotations and movements in opposite directions, and encases the body like a double helix. It has an impact on our posture, maintains balance at all levels, and ensures a precise forward directed course when walking. This line also generates rotations and stabilizes the body.

▥ Fascial Chains in Motion

In certain movements, the long fascial chains are even visible; they can be observed, for example, in javelin or discus throwing, in swinging movements, and in certain forms of gymnastics. These types of movement were formerly part of the health exercise culture, as historical images show, but today these poses look somewhat out of date.

Some of our fascia exercises resemble such swing exercises. Older sport doctrines and exercise forms used the long fascia chains more, but these have been somewhat forgotten in the modern science of exercising.

Anatomical illustrations of fascial chains compared with sports and gymnastics poses.

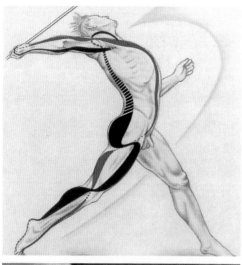

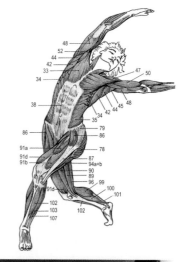

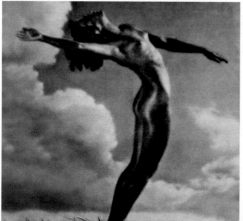

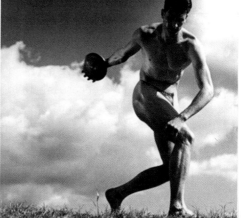

Gymnastics Old School

Our grandparents and great-grandparents knew about the dynamic exercises that focus on the long fascia strings, especially those which involve swinging, rhythmic, full-body movements that stimulate the entire body. This "physical education" was accessible to men and women in the 19th century, and became very popular between 1900 and 1950; people practiced with balls, tires, and clubs, which were swung or thrown. The participants stretched and bent themselves energetically in all directions.

Hinrich Medau— book title from 1940.

These gymnastic forms have a long tradition and include elements from dance, medical exercises, and coordination sports, such as fencing. The dancer Rudolf von Laban (1879–1958) was a co-founder of one of the schools that taught these disciplines. Hinrich and Senta Medau, who were music and gym teachers, founded a school that taught dance, full-body stretching, and swinging motions in the 1920s.

The old-fashioned-looking exercises clearly trigger the long fascia strings and utilize the elastic recoil capacity of these collagenous tissues rather than relying on muscular effort. While the former teachers were choosing these movements for their aesthetic elegance, it is only due to the recent insights from the field of fascia research that we now understand how specifically this 'elegance' is achieved.

HOW DOES CONNECTIVE TISSUE RESPOND TO TRAINING?

The fascia is alive—it responds to stimuli and adapts to mechanical stretch loading. Therefore, if stimulated by targeted and regular training, it slowly but sustainably adapts its tissue architecture. The fact that the elastic and resilient qualities improve as a result of training has been demonstrated in scientific experiments. If you do not move, you will become stiffer.

Fascial tissue degenerates if it is not exercised. Remember the "Use it or lose it" adage; this biological principle mentioned earlier also applies to the fascia. Photographs from Japanese researchers show that the fascia becomes acutely matted and clotted after a period of immobility; it loses its regular lattice-like architecture. This matting affects the functioning of the muscles, because the fiber bundles cannot properly slide against each other, the power transmission from muscle to muscle no longer works smoothly, and coordination suffers.

Because of the matting, the flow of movement is hindered and more energy is required; posture also suffers and stiffness will be felt, because the matted tissue is less elastic. It is now known that back pain patients have clotted, matted lumber fascia. Matted or clogged fascial tissue is also a symptom of old age; young people have

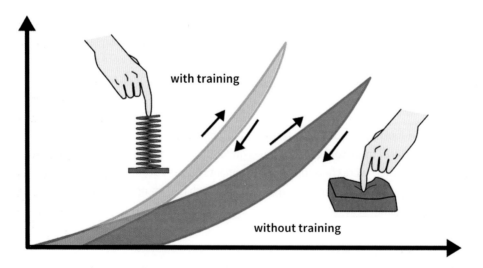

In the case of trained animals, the tissue is deformed under loading and will rapidly bounce back without much delay. The tissue of untrained animals, on the other hand, bounces back with a significant delay; it loses more energy on its return.

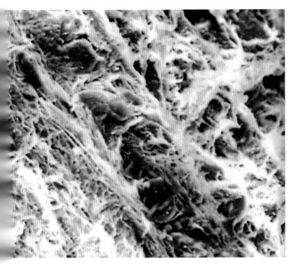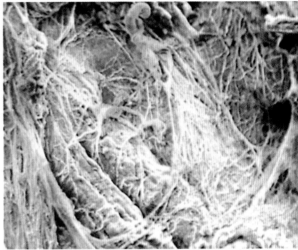

Normal fascial tissue in a healthy body (left). Fascia in a body part that has been immobilized in a plaster cast for several weeks (right).

an even, regular tissue structure, while the fascia of the elderly (who are less active) tends to be tangled and matted together, thus losing its regular wavy structure.

Some of these phenomena are probably natural, because the connective tissue cells produce more collagen when aging; in addition the exchange and removal of old fiber occurs more slowly, the tissue does not get renewed as dynamically as before, and there is less water in the matrix. Exercising is therefore a very good way to address these symptoms, in order to decelerate the process; the cells are encouraged to produce new collagen, and the decomposition of old collagen is accelerated.

A similar tendency has long been known in muscular research: as we age, the muscles normally tend to waste away, but through exercise this process can be halted. Even among seniors, lost muscle mass can be rebuilt. This is why the fascia can work well into old age—we can still keep our fascia firm, elastic, and healthy by exercising. The more the fascia is mobilized and trained in the right way, the longer it will work for us.

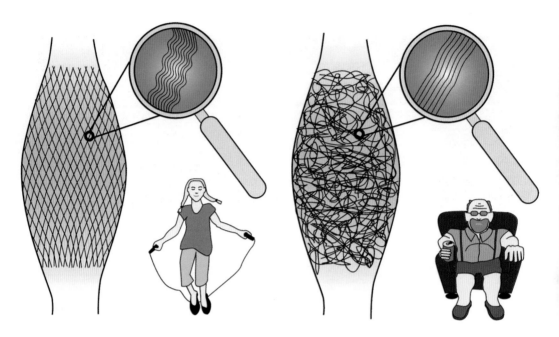

In older people, (right), the fascia entangles and loses its elasticity not only as a result of aging, but also because of less activity.

▦ Fascia Training Acts with Time

Fascia responds to exercising, but not in the same way as muscles. The metabolic turnover rate of fascia is not as high as that of muscles: the natural process of continuous replacement of connective tissue fibers is slower than that of muscle tissue. However, when the connective tissue cells receive the right stimuli, they become more agile and tend to produce fibers, which form a regular lattice-oriented network and reveal the typical wavy alignment as in young people whose bodies are better adapted to elastic recoil movements such as in rope-skipping, bouncing or dancing. The architecture of the fascia adapts to regular stretch-loading demands—it changes its length, strength, and alignment. If tensile forces are frequently repeated, the collagenous fibers are strengthened and become more injury resistant. This is accompanied by a significantly higher elastic capacitance—in other words, a greater capacity to act as a spring. Even when the fabric has been neglected and not been sufficiently loaded for several days or weeks, perhaps because of a temporary period of sickness, a renewed training program can once again stimulate the tangled tissue.

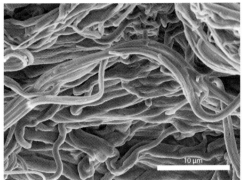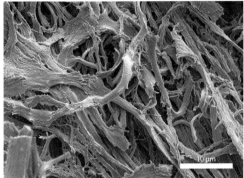

Young and old: comparison of the fibers of a 6-year-old child (left) and a 90-year-old person (right).

We know from studies of athletes, runners, and tennis players how well the fascia adapts to tension. Athletes of most disciplines tense their muscles and joints in starting and stopping movements, which hardens and tightens their lateral muscles. The surrounding fascia, the fascia lata, located on the outside of the thigh, flattens the form of the thigh on the outside, as seen from the front. This occurs through the normal stress of walking, even with non-athletes. We examined this by measuring the thigh fascia of wheelchair users: their fascia is much thinner than that of people who can walk, but do not exercise. The situation is different in professional riders, however, because riders load the muscles on the inside of the thigh more strongly—the adductors; as a result, the fascia here becomes very strong. This sometimes leads to the expression of a so-called 'rider's bone' within the adductor fascia; due to the heavy loading there. While most riders do not develop this pathological ossification, this tissue adaptation is found as frequently in inner thighs of professional riders as the typical heel spur is found in the plantar fascia of normal walking people.

■ Sports Injuries, Especially to the Fascia

For athletes in particular, who want to avoid injuries, the state of the fascia network is vitally important. If a football player is hobbling to the edge of the field in pain (or has to be taken off the field), if a tennis player withdraws because of shoulder pain, or if a runner pulls out shortly after the start of a race, it is usually because of a weakness in fascial tissues: the ligaments, tendons, muscle fascia, or joint capsules will usually suffer from sprains, tears, or micro injuries. In most cases, these fascial injuries occur

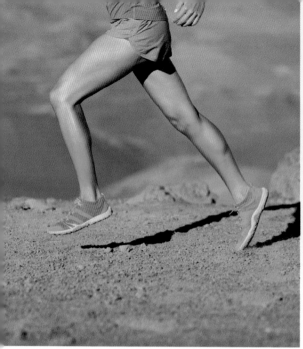

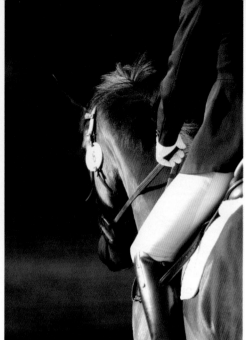

Runners and tennis players have a very robust outer fascia lata.

Riders sit firmly on horseback, which strengthens the fascia of the inner thigh.

as a result of the body being subjected to a level of strain that it is not strong enough to tolerate, or because the particular region has suffered an injury in the past. Such strenuous injuries occur most commonly to the white collagenous fibers within the soft tissues, i.e. the fascia, and not to the red muscle fibers. This means, that in most athletes, their fascial components are the weakest links, not their bones or their muscle fibers. Even in so-called muscle tears, it is rarely the muscle fibers themselves which are torn, rather than their fascial extensions.

Specific fascia training can therefore protect athletes against injury. Because healthy fascia can store and release more kinetic energy, it becomes stronger when subjected to strain, develops more elastic resilience, and also heals faster.

▥ News About Sore Muscles

In connection with regeneration after training and exercise, fascia research has shed new light on a phenomenon that has so far baffled us, even though it is so common: the form of muscle ache which is known as delayed onset muscle soreness. This occurs regularly after excessive or unfamiliar activities, particularly after eccentric movements, such as when walking downhill. The period of most soreness is usually not observed on the same day, but one or few days afterwards.

Various explanations have been put forward over the years: too much lactic acid that leaves agitating crystals in the muscles; inflammation caused by free radicals; metabolic factors; cramps; or tears in the muscle fibers. However, all these theories have so far not been able to fully explain the phenomenon.

The lactic acid theory was accepted for a long time, but has been proved insufficient, since it became clear that this form of muscle ache also occurs even when little lactate is produced. In addition, the amount of lactate in the body is reduced by half after about 20 minutes, whereas the muscle ache tends to last for a day or more.

The hypothesis of tears in the muscles is still predominant in conventional teaching of the science of exercise. This leads to the belief that it is not recommended to massage sore muscles, as the tears are seen as fresh injuries, and the massage would therefore reinforce the pain. It is thought that these tears occur in the muscle fibers, followed by mild edema and inflammation. The origin of this hypothesis is a classic test developed by Scandinavian anatomists: they allow

Tennis player Tommy Haas was forced to leave the court at the French Open in spring 2014 because of overstretched tendons in his shoulder. In professional tennis, impact forces can reach speeds of up to 230 km/h, which the shoulder has to absorb.

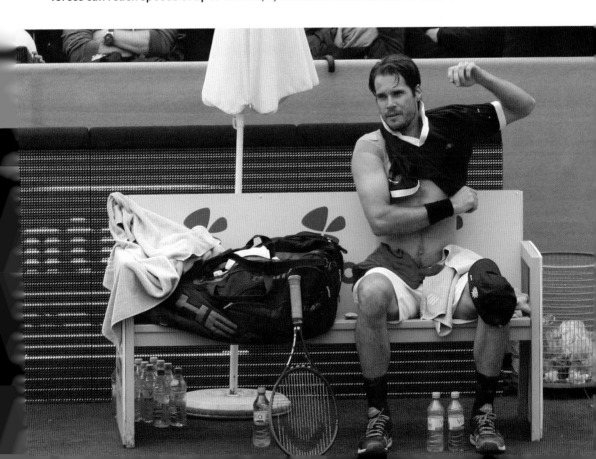

subjects to repeatedly step onto a chair with the same leg and step down again in such a way that the other leg gets loaded in order to selectively trigger muscle soreness. In the descending leg that has to brake heavily in downwards stepping, the subjects indeed developed a muscle ache.

The anatomists took tissue samples and analyzed them under an electron microscope; they found that there were definitely changes to the muscle fibers, in their smallest units—the sarcomeres. However, this could be documented only in very extreme and non-physiological loading protocols.

However, new studies have now shifted the focus on the fascial components. Recent studies have shown that the fascial sheath of the muscle—the epimysium—is evidently the main source of the sensation of pain in sore muscles. The early history of this new discovery can be traced back to a congress in 2007, when I sat on the podium along with some pain and muscle researchers. We discussed a planned study that aimed to explore muscle soreness.

The researchers wanted to inject a saline solution into the muscles of subjects suffering from muscle ache, in order to pinpoint the local origin of the soreness. The test with saline solution is an accepted procedure in pain research. In wounds and inflammation, the brine increases the pain locally and therefore indicates where the sensitive nerve

endings are located which are the origin of the pain.

After we had talked about the role of fascia, Thomas Graven-Nielsen, a Danish pain researcher, modified the experimental set-up. As in the case of the classic experiment with the chair, he and his colleague William Gibson, an Australian physiotherapy expert, triggered delayed onset muscle soreness in a group of subjects with the Scandinavian stair stepping protocol described before. Subsequently they waited a day and then injected the saline solution in both legs either into the muscle belly on the thigh or into the fascial envelope around this same muscle. While there was hardly any sensitive reaction from the injections in the upwards-walking leg, in the downward walking leg the injection detected a very sensitive pain response from the fascial envelopes, and not from the muscle belly. Interestingly, the test subjects could not differentiate whether their pain came from the red muscle or the fascia; they just felt "the muscle hurt." Later the researchers repeated these tests with several other muscles and different kinds of stimulation; and found the same response: the fascial envelope – rather than the inside muscle fibers themselves – seems to be the tissue where the muscle soreness sensation originates.

While this new finding caused a sensation within the field of sports science in 2009, it is still unclear whether delayed onset muscle soreness occurs because of tears, edema, or inflammation in the fascial envelopes themselves —or whether the sensitization of nerve endings in the fascia is triggered by other processes, such as injuries or inflammatory processes inside the muscle. In any case, the sensitization of the fascial envelope serves as the primary origin of the soreness, not the muscle fibers underneath.

After a few days the pain will go away by itself and the fascia will have regained its normal tolerance. Clearly, the fascia adapts to any new strain to which it is subjected; this also protects against new muscle soreness.

You can find more on this below, in the training principles, as well as in the exercises in Chapter 3. For now we can say that the new-found knowledge of fascia participation has changed both the theory and the treatment options for sore muscles—and has implications for the prevention of this soreness. Healthy and fit fascia is less prone to muscle ache, which is a good reason for selective training.

Goals of Fascia Training

We are training for:

- Optimum energy storage capacity

- Ideal elastic extensibility and tension

- Smooth functioning of the long fascia chains

- Youthful wave structure of the fascia

- Rapid regeneration of the muscle fascia unit after strain

WHAT YOU SHOULD KNOW ABOUT FASCIA TRAINING

Fascia training is not the same as muscle training. Many muscle exercises in conventional programs move and exercise the fascia to some degree automatically; however, this is not the case with all programs—and not for all types of fascial tissue. Additionally, muscle fascia needs specific impulses, in order to respond optimally. Many common training programs are geared primarily toward increasing muscular strength or cardiovascular conditioning, but the specific loading responses of fascial tissue are not as well emphasized. The particular impulses that fascia and tendons need, especially for rebuilding, regeneration, or fluid exchange, cannot simply be achieved in an optimal manner by pressing weights or by performing unilateral exercises.

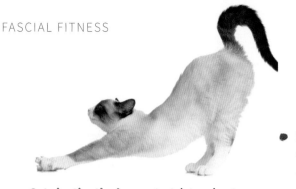

Cats instinctively use stretch tension to activate their muscles and fascia; the stretching is not passive but active with often simultaneous muscular activation.

For many athletes, such as dancers, gymnasts, wrestlers, and other sportspersons, a comprehensive range of free mobility is very important: they need strength, flexibility, and good all-round full-body coordination. Because they protect against injury and facilitate normal activities, everyday mobility and good coordination must be a target.

▦ How to Reach the Fascia in Training

As studies have shown, strength training and regular exercises do not necessarily train the body-wide fascial net in a sufficient manner. One reason for this is the arrangement of the fibers in the fascia in relation to the muscles. Fascia are structured as plates or cases around the different muscles, and their fibers run in different directions:

- parallel to the muscle direction

- transversely to the muscle direction

- in a serial – i.e. straight line – alignment with the muscle fibers; which usually is the case at the tendons

The parallel-running muscle fibers will not be affected or trained using normal weight training; the specific fibers in question here are located e.g. in the perimysium and epimysium—the connective tissue around the muscle fiber cases. These fibers need stimulation during training, in order to encourage their metabolism and to ensure that they are suitably trained.

This is achieved using stretches in which the whole muscle unit is elongated. By means of melting stretches, in which the muscle fibers are both relaxed and elongated at the same time, we can reach deeper muscle and fascia segments than with regular muscular exercise contractions. These melting stretches therefore form part of our training program.

Additionally, there is the combination of stretching and muscle contraction; this means that we sometimes tense the elongated muscles during an external resistance when stretching—like a stretching cat that sometimes enjoys to pull back its claws against the resistance of the floor (or leather couch) when arriving at the longest stretch position.

Not Automatic: Muscle and Fascia Training

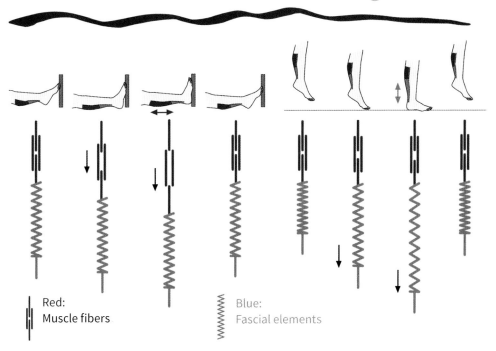

Red:
Muscle fibers

Blue:
Fascial elements

Look at the left four illustrations. Here the calf muscles are trained using conventional exercises: pushing a plate away from you with your feet, which is a classic power exercise. The red elements in the diagram are the contractile muscle fibers, which change in length during exercise. The blue springs symbolize the elastic (fascial) structures; these do not change significantly in their length, and are thus not very well stimulated by this type of workout.

The right four illustrations are different. Here the exercise uses elastic recoil motions, such as hopping or jumping actions. Here it is the tendinous elements—the blue spring elements—which change their length the most; in this case it is the Achilles tendon which receives the appropriate training stimulus.

The Achilles tendon changes like an elastic yo-yo; it elongates under tension and then recoils rapidly in the subsequent dynamic power movement. The muscular fibers on the other side mainly serve as impulse control gadgets and change their length only minimally.

Stretching and Training: What the Fascia Needs

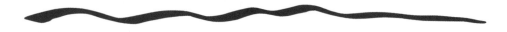

The images below show what happens to the fascia when a muscle is subjected to various activities and stress. First of all, the inside of the muscle—the blue elements in the diagram—represent the fascia and the fibers running round the muscle inside and the muscle in specific directions.

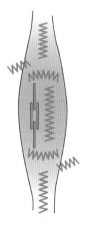

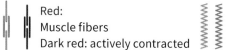

Red:
Muscle fibers
Dark red: actively contracted

Blue:
Fascial elements
Dark blue: stretch-loaded

Here we see the muscle and fascia fibers at rest: there are longitudinal, transverse, and serially arranged fascial elements, shown here in blue. The red muscle fibers are relaxed, and so are all the fascial elements.

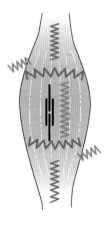

During a classical muscle strength exercise, the muscle shape changes. Note the blue elements in this example of the biceps muscle: if you hold a dumbbell in your hand and raise it, so that the elbow bends, the muscle fibers inside the biceps muscle contract and shorten. This results in an increase of the biceps diameter; it widens. This induces an elongation and stretch stimulation of the blue fascia elements which run transverse to the main muscle fibers. In addition, the fascial elements in the tendon areas are stretch loaded as they are elongated by the muscular contraction.

So far, so good. The fascial elements which run parallel to the muscle fibers, however, are not being elongated and are therefore not stretch-loaded. These elements are within the perimysium and the endomysium—the intramuscular connective tissues which surround the muscle fibers and muscle fiber bundles. Therefore these parallel oriented fascial elements do not get sufficiently 'trained' in this mode of exercise.

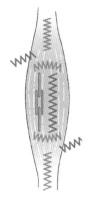

Melting stretch, as in normal passive stretching. Here the muscle shape is elongated, but does not become thicker, since the red muscle fibers do not actively contract. In fact, the red muscle fibers are passively relaxed and elongated. Thus these pink muscle fibers are limp; but the fascial elements which run parallel to the muscle are elongated and stretch-loaded. Nevertheless, a similar elongation does not occur at the fascial elements in the tendon areas, as these are arranged in series with the pink (limp) muscle fibers.

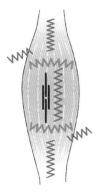

Active resistance stretch: here the muscle fibers are actively contracted against an external resistance while the whole muscle unit is in an elongated (stretched) condition. Note that almost all fascial segments are stretch-loaded and therefore stimulated in this modality. If one were forced to practice one stretching modality only, this one would therefore be the most comprehensive. An alternation with the two previously shown exercise modalities would, however, ensure an even better inclusion of all fascial elements within and around the muscle.

The exercises in our program take into consideration the various effects of muscle strength, passive stretching, and active stretching stress, and this is achieved in many different ways. In so doing, we are able to reach the different fascial tissue components, which are present in various arrangements in and around the muscle.

▥ Features of Healthy Fascia and Good Training

The goal of our fascia training is therefore a fully functional fascial network throughout the whole body. From everything we have seen so far, the characteristics of healthy, well-trained fascia can be identified as follows:

1. It is firm and elastic at the same time.

2. It is flexible like bamboo.

3. It has the tensile strength of a rope.

4. It enables springy resilient movements similar to those of a gazelle.

Fascia training:

- Increases the resilient strength of tendons and ligaments;

- Avoids painful frictions in the hip joints and spinal discs;

- Protects a muscle from injury;

- Maintains a youthful body shape, with a well-toned muscle definition and body contour.

The advantages of a fit fascia for engaging in sports, but also for everyday life, are self-evident:

- Muscles work more efficiently.

- Recovery times are considerably shortened, so you recuperate faster for the next workout and the next task.

- Performance increases.

- Movement and coordination improve.

- Long-term protection is provided against injury, pain, and disorders.

Injuries, disorders, and twisting and matting of the fascia are also involved in many other soft tissue complaints, including lower back pain, shoulder pain, elbow problems, neck pain, the dreaded plantar fasciosis (fasciitis), and so on. In all of these syndromes, the state of the connective tissue plays an important role; it may even be the single most important origin of the pathology — for example, in frozen shoulder conditions or in heel spur pain. Most of the problems mentioned above are signs that our fascia network reacts in an obstructive way when it is incorrectly exercised or is underutilized.

▥ What Is Man Made For?

We have all been amazed at what stunning feats circus acrobats, dancers, gymnasts, fencers, judo fighters, or extreme climbers on steep rock faces are capable of.

The human movement repertoire is extremely diverse, as in any other animal species. In fact, we are probably the only species that is capable of conscious, coordinated and highly complex movement orchestration with other individuals, such as in dancing.

Descended from tree dwellers that pulled themselves in swinging manner from branch to branch, we later advanced to walking upright on two legs, developing into dancers and runners whose performance is characterized by a high degree of economical endurance.

Accordingly, it stands to reason that natural movement for humans is marked by its wide versatility. However, we have something in common with other animals: our movements and walking partly contradict the fundamental principles of physics, the gravity of the earth and inertia of mass during rapid movement, which we have to respond to with every major motion. For my teacher Ida Rolf, the relationship of our body to gravity was an essential element around which she built her theory of body posture and movements.

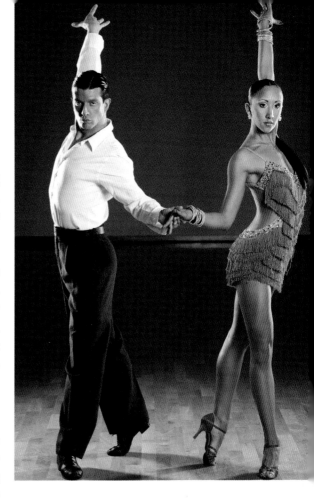

Unique coordination: people can coordinate their movements precisely with one another.

We are therefore, like most animals, built for confrontation with gravity, and specialists in versatility. If one or both of these elements is lacking, our organism reacts with degeneration and disease, because if the muscles do not receive the typical stress stimuli, then the bones and the fascia will start to break down and lose their strength, which can lead to pain and injury. Our modern way of life in the Western world underutilizes our body: we

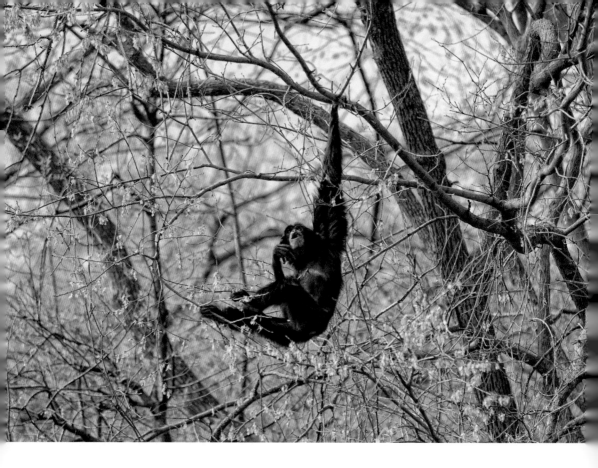

Chimpanzees move between the trees and the ground using very diverse movements.

train only a fraction of the possible range of motion appropriate to our species. Many people, especially with increasing age, do load their bodies inadequately.

We might think that we can allow certain skills to quietly dwindle because we no longer need them in the modern world. However, the Stone Age still lingers in our bones, as the medical scientist Detlev Ganten of the famous Charité Clinic in Berlin says:

We notice when something is lacking. Our body reacts to immobility, underuse, and incorrect strain with deficiency symptoms—sore joints, degenerated discs, arthritis, and inflammation, not to mention obesity, metabolic disorders, diabetes, and heart attacks. In addition, we cannot disregard the psychological aspect: lack of exercise and depression as well as some forms of dementia appear to be related to this deficiency. The awareness of how healthy movement affects the psyche and mental fitness is on the increase. We appreciate the concern about the consequences of the lack of movement; however, apart from generalities, there is a growing awareness of how important the correct forms of movement are. These whole-body movements include coordination and dexterity, balance, stimulation of the long fascial chains incorporating the larger functional units, and natural movement patterns.

Some researchers believe that only versatile, adequate demand on the musculoskeletal system guarantees health in the long term, as well as preventing arthritis and joint inflammation. Their theory is known as unused-arc theory, and it states that we do not load our joints sufficiently over the full available range that they were originally constructed for by natural selection and the evolution of our homo sapiens ancestors. Observations of the natural movements of our closest monkey relatives, such as chimpanzees, have provided us with facts about their typical movement patterns: the animals hang, climb, jump, and grab firmly, supporting their own weight; and they sit and crawl, while stretching, and challenging and using their joints over their full range of motion.

The impression of researchers is that both the upright posture of humans and the use of shoes, and sometimes the long periods of sitting during the daily work routine, lead to disorders, because the maximum strain and the natural range of stretching of our joints are restricted. This can lead to problems in the cartilage, such as arthritis in the fingers, which up to now has mainly been explained by excessive wear and tear. In fact, it seems to be more the insufficient loading of the joints—our inadequate and non-species-appropriate strain application to the joints—that is the cause. An example that supports this theory is the case of osteoarthritis.

Osteoarthritis of the hip joint begins in the underused areas, namely the edges, and then continues into the strained sites, such as the femoral head. It might originally not be wear and tear, but something quite different—the result of underuse of our evolutionary system, or the result of incorrect, non-species-appropriate movement. One consequence of these considerations is that physicians now increasingly recommend moving and stretching for osteoarthritis.

The success currently being experienced by climbing walls in hospitals and rehabilitation facilities confirms the unused-arc hypothesis. Climbing activates the evolutionary spectrum of our movement patterns and simultaneously uses many muscles and ligaments. This requisite coordination also involves arms-over-the-head movements and the shoulder and neck muscles. All this yields good results in pain relief, back problems, and healing after surgery, as well as success in neurological conditions, such as strokes, multiple sclerosis, and anxiety disorders.

Aside from clinics and disease, there is also a growing trend for everyday exercises and sport activities that match these findings—

in particular, playgrounds for adults. These outdoor areas consist of climbing walls and adventure courses, where even the elderly can playfully experiment with new body positions and movements which do not occur during their habitual everyday living activities. These are excellent new developments in our society, particularly from a fascial health perspective.

I go to a nearby park in Munich as often as I can, where a climbing net and some gym bars have been set up; I exercise outdoors, putting my body through all sorts of

Pensioners on the playground: the health benefits of this new trend are currently being scientifically investigated.

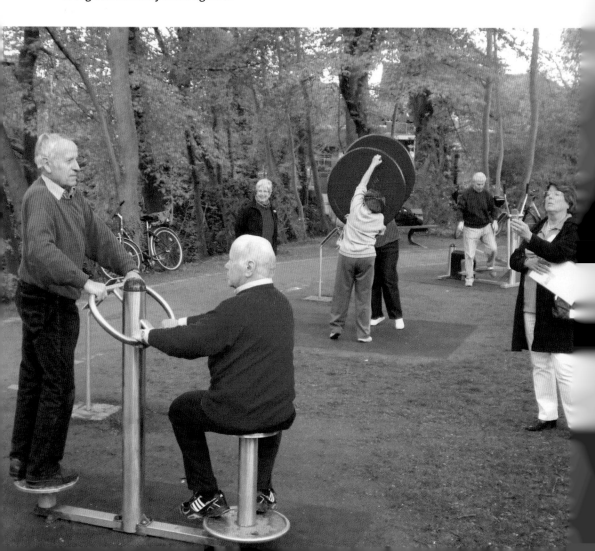

monkey-like contortions and swinging in different directions (see image on p. 86). After a long day in the laboratory or on the road, I do not know of anything better for recovering and refreshing than such playful monkey-gym explorations. When hanging upside down for brief periods of rest in between, one cannot resist laughing about the world around and about, oneself included.

■ The Right Stimuli for the Fascial Network

All the discussion presented above leads us to the conclusion that we need to combine different training stimuli. These different demands are necessary for the various fascia functions and the entire body-wide network, as well as for the maintenance and care of the tissue architecture. The fascia loves dynamic exercise and stretching, in addition to mechanical pressure and training. Mechanical pressing or rolling has the goal of refreshing liquid exchange. This will be dealt with later in the training program; briefly, rolling with balls or specially designed foam rollers may achieve such a desired effect. The fascia is squeezed like a sponge, with a resulting exchange of liquid. This acts as a kind of self-massage and can help with muscle pain and stiffness.

There is another important element to be considered: the stimulation of sensory functions in the fascia. As we now know, the fascia can be regarded as our richest sensory organ. Our movements are fundamentally dependent on our sensorial perception—particularly on the processing of information from the motion detectors in our fascia, our joints, skin and muscles. A fostering of the sensorial stimulation and a fine-tuning of the related perception within our body-wide connective tissue network must therefore be part of any fascia training. Playful sensations, well-being, and stimulation of our movement perception all improve sensory refinement—and the rate of success of training. Such a training orientation does not only increase the level of fun but also the overall benefit for our health.

A Brief Summary

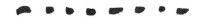

The training stimuli during fascia training include:

- Variety of movement

- Inclusion of moments of muscular activation

- High strain application for the engagement of elastic storage capacity

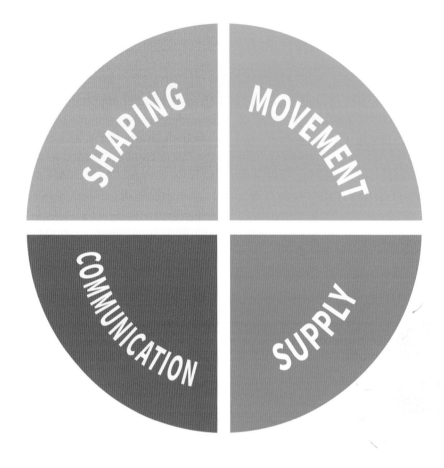

- Loading of the long functional fascial chains across several joints

- Activate species-appropriate natural movement patterns

- Respecting regeneration and remodeling times

- Gentle melting stretch stimulation and self-myofascial massage

- Sensory impulses and body awareness

THE FOUR DIMENSIONS OF A FASCIA WORKOUT

Our fascia training needs to be versatile; it is structured according to four principles, which correspond to the four basic functions, as introduced in Chapter 1 (see p. 26). For each of these four basic functions there are specifically tailored training impulses—the four dimensions of the fascia workout. If you compare the concepts with each other, each basic function is associated with a particular form of training:

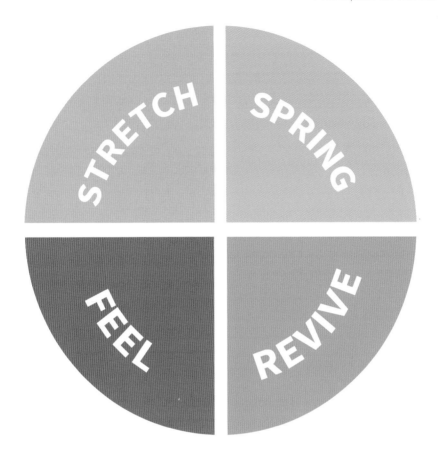

Function:
Shaping + Movement + Communication + Supply

Training:
Stretch + Spring + Feel + Revive

The image of the circle with a cross was not chosen by chance: the circle is evocative of the continuum—the four functions considered as a whole. The coordinated system in the middle shows the four different training dimensions that are necessary in order to reach the fascia tissue. They differ from each other and have to be considered individually.

All of them actually belong together, and all four should be exercised in order to ensure that all types of fascial tissue in the deeper layers and fibers are stimulated as well. The circle with the cross will guide you through the exercise chapter (Chapter 3) and serve as a teaching aid. It shows:

● Which exercise belongs to which function

- Which discomfort or problem needs to be addressed by which basic function

- What kind of training impulse must be applied

For this purpose, we have color highlighted the different areas using the respective terms. First, you should become familiar with how the basic functions are dealt with by the four dimensions.

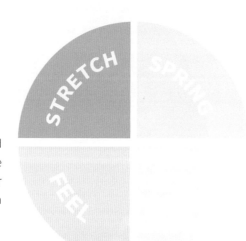

1. Stretch (Basic Function: Shaping)

Stretching is a natural strain and stimulates the mechanical qualities of the fascia, which is the shaping substance. Many kinds of movement, but stretching in particular, will activate the long fascial chains.

For centuries, stretching exercises have been part of training programs, especially for dancers and acrobats. Regular stretching can actually extend the range of motion and this includes not only the muscles but the joints as well; however, it can do a lot more, as discovered from years of research.

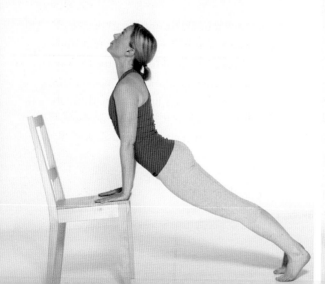

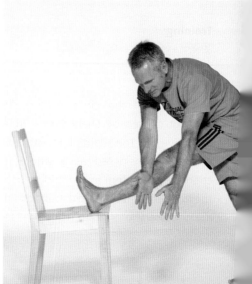

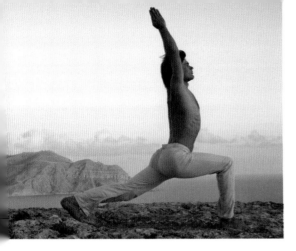

Yoga also acts on the fascia.

Yoga, which has experienced global success, is based on the stretching of fascial tissue. The slow, methodical stretching which is endured for long periods has a physiological impact: the blood pressure and the pulse are changed significantly— they both decrease. Therefore, when fascial tissue is stretched, signals are transmitted to the autonomic nervous system; this activates the parasympathetic nervous system, which is then followed by a relaxation response. The mystical effects of yoga in meditation and in the calming of stressed modern minds are essentially based on this fact.

But yoga does even more: it also acts on the fascia. Yoga can help people with back pain, and this has now been scientifically proved. An essential factor in this is the stretching component. An American study showed that back pain patients who did yoga stretching exercises achieved results that were as good as those for patients who completed a conventional back training program. This in turn has strengthened the reputation of yoga, which is now accepted by health insurance companies. To find out more, including details on these studies, see Chapter 4.

Stretching, however, has been caught in the crossfire of the theories of modern exercise science since the 1980s. While it had been recommended for decades as a form of injury protection when performed before sports, many sports scientists later questioned its protective effects and even cautioned against the use of static stretching before athletic performance. However, now the same scientists are partly paddling backwards since more and more studies do reveal some long-term tissue remodeling effects.

Today there are different types of stretching, including dynamic, ballistic stretching (for example, reaching to the floor with your fingertips and stretching in short bursts), and slow, long-duration, static stretching (carefully taking a stretch position and remaining there for a long time without rocking). From a fascial perspective, we use both forms of stretching: small elastic bounces in a stretched position, as well as slow static stretching. They each serve a different purpose and support various physiological connective tissue types. We do not consider the exclusive stretching of isolated, individual muscles as very effective. In contrast, the exercises in our program take the form of a playful, creative full-body workout and specific stretching for longer myofascial chains. These are simple exercises, including small modifications of known stretching exercises, with which one can optimally stimulate the whole muscle-fascia system.

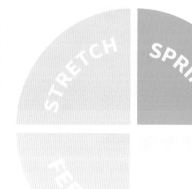

2. Spring (Basic Function: Movement)

Springing exercises, such as jumping or swinging the upper body, stimulate the elastic storage capacity within the fascia, which is important for basic movement functions. This generally applies to all muscular fascia tissues, but especially to the tendinous portions. The principle of storage and release of tensile energy is applied in all exercises of this kind, as they involve elastic recoil motions.

One variant is the preparatory countermovement in which the tendons and fascia are extended and loaded with tensile power, similarly to when a javelin thrower extends back. This tension increase is an important factor in everyday movements:

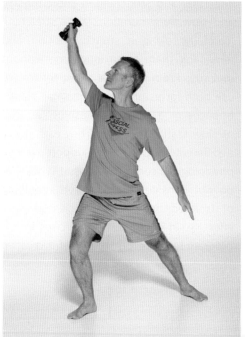
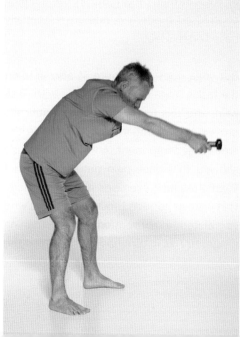

bending and getting back up, and lifting light or heavier objects, are based on the regulation of preparatory tension in the fascia. Full-body spring exercises stimulate the long fascial chains; if you exercise in all directions, these long chains will be included.

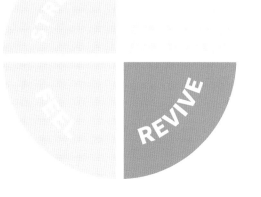

3. Revive (Basic Function: Supply)

The reviving of the fascia in our program takes place through a kind of self-massage. Foam rollers are commercially available for this, but alternatively other tools such as tennis or rubber balls can be used.

In all of these exercises, mechanical pressure and shear motion are applied to the connective tissue; this simply leads to a liquid exchange in the fascia. The tissue is literally squeezed like a sponge, transporting metabolites and lymph away, and then partly refills with new and fresh water from the blood plasma in the small capillaries. This exchange stimulates the metabolism and improves fluid supply to the fascia, but also to associated organs, thereby invigorating and regenerating the fascia.

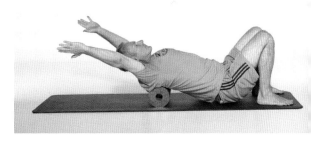

The fluid renewal effect can be achieved using various manual physiotherapy techniques. Fascia loves pressure, specifically an optimum therapeutic dose of variable pressure, as if wringing or squeezing a sponge. It reacts particularly well to the application of this persistent, slow, gentle pressure application. We use such techniques in Rolfing; treatments such as myofascial release and many osteopathic techniques also use the same effect. As we found out in Chapter 1, pressure also triggers a cascade of signals toward the autonomic nervous system and in the direction of our muscles. The right amount of pressure reduces fascial and muscle tightness, so that tension and adhesions can be resolved.

The massaging and invigorating exercises in our fascia training rejuvenate the tissue; the result is not only a refreshed body but also one that is significantly more mobile. There is now a rapidly growing market for such fascial treatments using pressure, such as self-myofascial massage, blackroll training, MELT method, FasciaReleazer, the ROLL model, and many more. The exercises with a foam roller shown in this book can be used in a daily training regime, and also as a quick self-treatment, because they can release tension and alleviate pain and soreness.

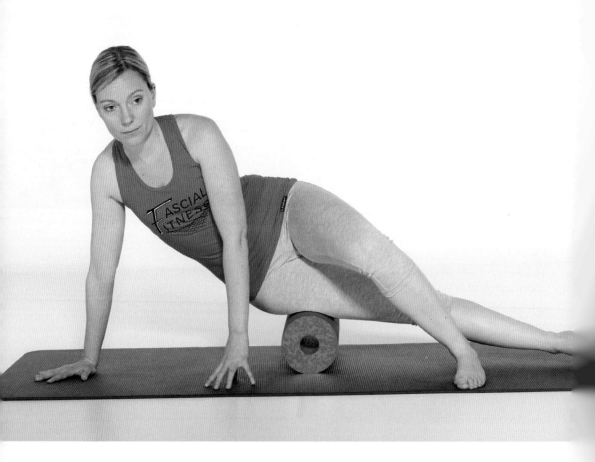

4. Feel (Basic Function: Communication)

The perception of body motion is extremely important for all movements and for the brain, as we have seen in Chapter 1. In movement science, but also in psychology, this body perception and its effect on the body image in the brain are now considered to be fundamentally important. The perceptual quality of movement has great importance, especially from the viewpoint of increasing physical inactivity in modern life. It clearly also plays a major role in many neurological and also psychological diseases. There is a lot of research literature under the general topic of embodied cognitive science.

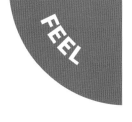

In fascia training we stimulate body perceptions via sensory impulses and exercises that raise your body awareness. Small movements—subtle changes in the location or in the direction on which you are focused—help you to appreciate perceptual nuances and to explore them with a spirit of curious discovery. This sensitivity occurs in a variety of exercises, which are fun oriented, so that you enjoy the exercises with your body. All this will—via the fascia—heighten the fine-tuning of your movement perception and coordination, and improve your total agility and fitness.

Important note: Avoid becoming distracted during practice. Keep your mindful attention oriented to your body; only then will there be a benefit that registers in your brain. In this way, lasting changes will be achieved by your training.

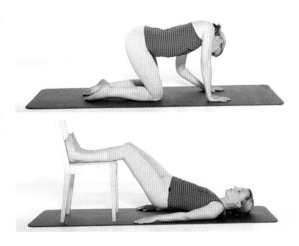

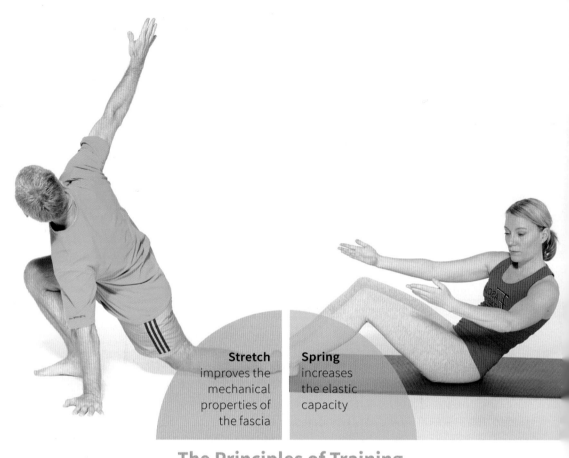

Stretch
improves the
mechanical
properties of
the fascia

Spring
increases
the elastic
capacity

The Principles of Training

Feel
stimulates
and refines
the body
perception

Revive
regenerates
the tissue
through fluid
exchange

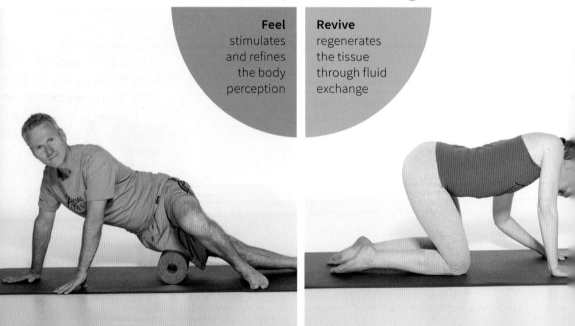

BEFORE WE START: WHAT CONNECTIVE TISSUE TYPE ARE YOU?

After discussing the theoretical foundations and principles, I am sure you will be keen to finally get started. Here is a short test which I invite you to do before you start practicing the exercises.

Assess the basic type of your connective tissue. This test will be useful, because there is a whole range of connective tissue types which all occur naturally. The two ends along a continuous spectrum constitute two poles: (1) people with firm, strong tissue; and (2) those with naturally very loose, soft connective tissue. Some connective tissue types are prone to develop typical weaknesses or hurdles during training, and not all exercises are appropriate for all types.

The two opposite poles may be described as:

- Viking type: firm connective tissue—strong and compact type with a high degree of stability and lack of flexibility.

- Flexible dancer type: loose, soft tissue—more delicate, more flexible type, such as is frequently found in contortionists, in Indian temple dancers or circus artists.

Both variants are normal, with equal frequency of occurrence. Men are more frequently found on the Vikings side, whereas women are more prone for the types with soft connective tissue. This tendency is due to physiological differences between the sexes:

- Men have more muscle mass; they have stronger muscles as well as stiffer muscular connective tissues.

- The collagen fibers in the subcutaneous fat of men are more tightly arranged than that of women.

- Women tend to have looser connective tissue, since (among other things) joint stiffness needs to change for pregnancy and childbirth.

- Women store different types of fat, and more of it, in the subcutaneous layers than men; this is a natural mechanism that acts as a reserve for pregnancy and lactating.

However, there are also Viking women, who have firmer connective tissues; likewise, there are also many men who are very mobile or dancer like. We know that, in most cases, the state of a person being much more flexible than average develops from early childhood. The girls and boys who are flexible by nature can easily do the splits, whereas the less flexible have to practice and might never succeed. Ballerinas and gymnasts mostly belong to the flexible type, although they also need a lot of muscle power as well.

Among men, the Viking types are often those whose external shape is more stability oriented ('like Obelix') and who are good at carrying heavy weights. Hyperflexible men on the other side are more likely to be dancers, gymnasts, and acrobats. However, there is a natural continuum here—some individuals are relatively close to one extreme, while other body types are more oriented in the middle.

Both connective tissue types are susceptible to specific symptoms. The flexible dancer types with soft connective tissue usually are prone to develop cellulite, herniated discs, and stretch marks after pregnancy. Strong connective tissue types, who we refer to as Vikings, often suffer Achilles tendon ruptures, and tend to have more severe scarring after wounds.

In the hands, problems with connective tissue can lead to deformation of the fingers. This disease, although usually benign, can be quite unpleasant; it is classified as a form of *fibromatosis*, a contracture of the connective tissue. The underlying cause is clearly a badly managed collagen synthesis in the fascia, and the myofibroblasts (the cells in the connective tissue that can close and wound and contract) are more active.

Men are two to eight times as likely to be affected by this fascial contracture as women. Viking types have more shoulder problems, such as stiffness or frozen shoulder. Parallel to the hand syndrome mentioned above, connective nodes and stiffness are common in the feet, medically termed as *plantar fibromatosis (fasciitis)*—this also occurs in Viking types more often than in average or in flexible dancer types.

As you can see, the advantages and disadvantages of both types are quite evenly distributed. For individuals at either pole of the tissue spectrum, namely Vikings and dancer types, different styles of training are recommended. We therefore have specific notes for both types in the exercise chapter.

You can now do the self-test to see where you stand: Test A is valid for everyone. After taking the test you will know which category you are in. However, if you only manage to achieve a few points, you should then do the additional Viking test. As this Viking test shows, many people are mixed types, with an average connective tissue quality, and are only locally stiff. They are reasonably mobile, usually do not get cellulitis that easily, can train to become very agile, and with regular practice can even do the splits.

Flexible Dancer Type

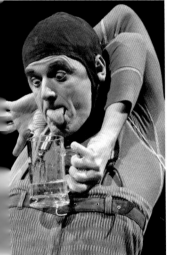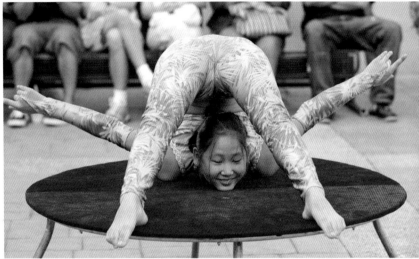

The contortionist and comedian Barto.

The young Mongolian contortionist dancer Enkhmurumhat commenced her training at the age of six.

Contortionists, acrobatic athletes and hyperflexible dancers usually train their mobility from childhood; in particular, they increase the range of motion of their joints and systematically stretch their connective tissues. Thanks to this type of training they are extremely mobile and can place their bodies into extraordinary positions. In circuses they are marveled at, and this contortionist "education" is traditional in Eastern circus schools, especially in Asia.

The majority of flexible dancer types are women. These types are inherently more mobile than other people. Nevertheless, they usually do not suffer from a pathological hypermobility syndrome (Marfan or Ehlers-Danlos syndromes), with inherited defective connective tissue.

The Self-Test: Determine Your Connective Tissue Type

Test A: Are You a Flexible Dancer Type?

● Can you bend with straight knees and place both palms flat on the ground? 1 point.

● Can you not only straighten your elbow joint, but extend it even further? Per arm: 1 point.

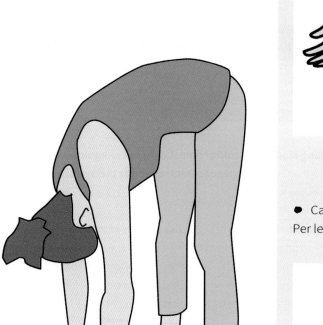

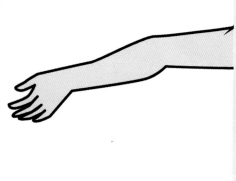

● Can you hyperextend your knee joint? Per leg: 1 point.

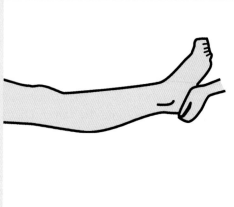

• Can you bend your thumb backward until it touches the forearm? Per hand: 1 point.

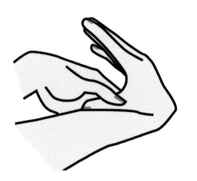

• Can you bend your little finger more than 90 degrees backward, toward the forearm? Per hand: 1 point.

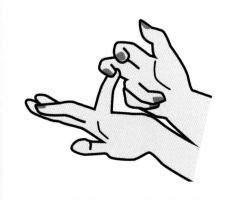

Evaluation

The maximum score is 9 points.

Score 6 or more points: you are most likely to be a flexible dancer type, with a genetic tendency for soft, pliable connective tissue.

In case you have achieved less than 6 points, we recommend you now perform also the following Viking test (Test B). And in case you have achieved only two or less points in this Test A, you are entitled to enter Test B with a 'bonus' of 3 Viking points.

Test B: Are You a Viking Type?

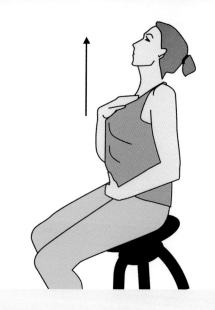

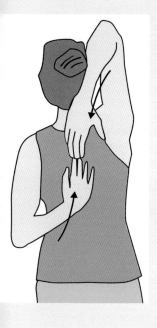

• If you try to join your hands behind your back (either with the right hand above or below), and the minimum distance of your hands is more than one hand lengths: 1 Viking point.

• Sit up straight on a chair without leaning on the backrest. Place one hand on the lower abdomen, with your thumb in front of the navel, and the other hand on your sternum. Without moving your lower abdomen and your bottom hand, now try to stretch your breastbone and your top hand upward, away from your bottom hand as far as possible. If you cannot achieve more than one hand width of movement in this stretching motion: 1 Viking point.

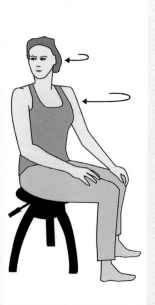

• Sit on a chair without leaning on the backrest. Turn your entire upper body and head as far as possible to the right and then to the left, while your pelvis and legs remain stable. If you cannot turn to 90 degrees or more in either direction: 1 Viking point.

• Stand up, with the knees extended, and bend forward in order to get your fingers as close to touch the ground as possible. If the minimal distance between your fingertips and the floor is one hand-length or more: 1 Viking point.

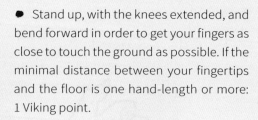
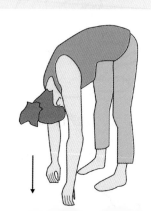

● Sit on the floor in a straddle position. If you can get your legs apart no more than 50 degrees: 1 Viking point.

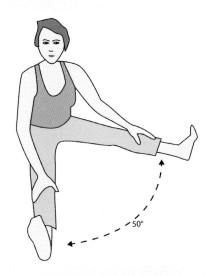

● While sitting, try to touch your forehead to each knee by lifting your leg and leaning forward accordingly. If you can touch neither your right knee nor your left knee with your forehead: 1 Viking point.

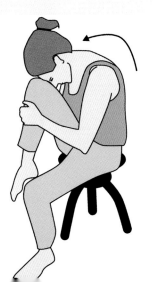

Depending on your age and sex, you may now deduct the following Viking points. If you are:

Male and over 35: deduct 2 points

Male and 35 or under: deduct 1 point

Female and over 35: deduct 1 point

Female and 35 or under: deduct 0 points.

Evaluation

5–9 points:

you are most likely a Viking type with a genetic disposition for an increased joint stability and less flexible connective tissues.

3–4 points:

you have limited mobility and are closer to the Viking type, but a genetic Viking makeup is not clearly identifiable. Your training condition and your lifestyle are probably influencing your flexibility to a similar degree as your genetic makeup.

1–2 points:

you have only local stiffness, but your general makeup is not the typical Viking type. You probably lie somewhere in the range of normal (i.e. average) flexibility in our Western society.

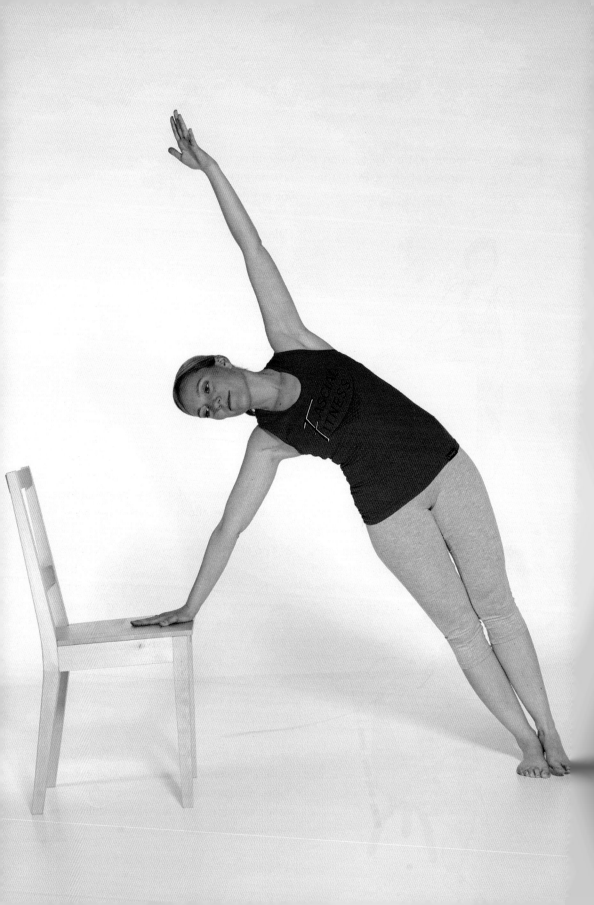

CHAPTER 3

The Exercises

Finally—the exercises! Now that you have battled through the long chapter of theory, it is time for the practice. Our fascial fitness exercise program is split up into several sections:

- A 10-minute training program—the basic program

- Exercises for problem areas: back, neck, arms, hips, and feet

- Notes for different connective tissue types—Vikings and Dancers

- Exercises of interest to both women and men

- Tips for athletes

- Tips for fascia-friendly, creative movements

- Fascia training in older age

This chapter presents descriptions of exercises using our two Fascial Fitness Trainers Daniela Meinl and Markus Rossmann as advisors and also as photographic models. All the exercises are drawn from the program of the Fascial Fitness Association (see the Appendix for more information and links to the website).

The basic training program consists of six exercises that cover the most important fascial chains. You should start gradually and do the program twice a week. Since it only takes about 10 minutes, you could integrate it into your existing fitness program or use the exercises as a warm-up. The other exercises you are welcome to practice additionally on an individual basis, depending on your interests or areas of concern.

In general, it is important to keep in mind the complete fascial web as a body-wide tensional network. This system cannot

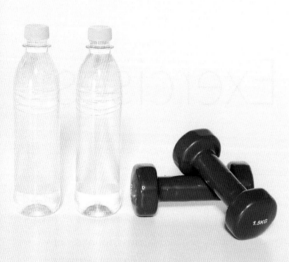

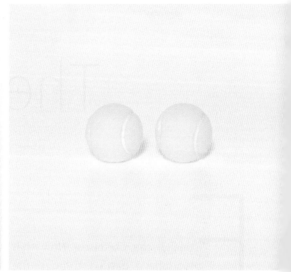

Small water bottles (500 ml) filled with tap water can be used instead of dumbbells.

Everyday tennis balls.

actually be trained in terms of localized areas only or as isolated parts of the body. All the exercises are aimed to influence the whole tensional network system. If you practice the basic program twice a week, and maybe add some of the additional exercises sporadically, then you will train your fascial net holistically and you will achieve the full benefits of this training program.

WHAT YOU WILL NEED

For some exercises you need a small, sturdy footstool, which should be approximately 20 to 30 cm in height. As an alternative, the exercises can be performed on a staircase step.

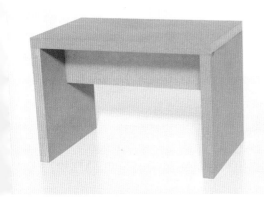

For some exercises you need a small, sturdy footstool, which should be approximately 20 to 30 cm in height. As an alternative, the exercises can be performed on a staircase step.

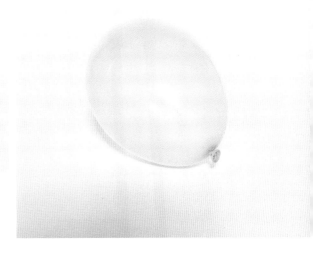

Balloon, inflated.

You can perform almost all of the exercises satisfactorily using everyday objects, which means you will not need to buy new equipment when you start the program. However, there is one exception: you will need a special foam roll, which is widely available from sports shops. We recommend that you obtain a foam roll specifically for fascia training, because it is difficult to substitute something else for one of these. There are several versions available; for guidance, you can check the Internet reference source in the Appendix. It is basically a hard foam roller, and common names for it are Blackroll, blueroll, fascia roll, or Pilates roll. As a beginner, it is best to start with a medium level of hardness. If in doubt, choose a roll on which you could perform the exercise '1. Rolling Out the Lumbar Fascia' (page 128) with a firm pressure feeling but no sharp pain sensations involved.

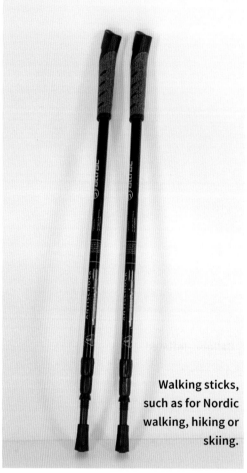

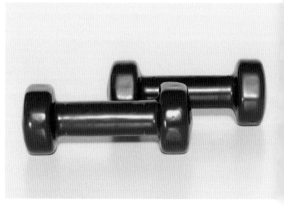

Small free weights, ranging from 0.5 kg to 1.5 kg.

Walking sticks, such as for Nordic walking, hiking or skiing.

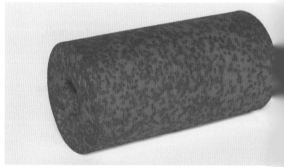

Medium foam roller.

If you plan to exercise regularly, there are some other items that may prove useful, all of which are available from sports shops:

CLOTHING AND SHOES

You can train in regular sports clothes or in yoga attire, or in a T-shirt and sweatpants or leggings. Whichever you choose, the material should be stretchy, comfortable, and sports-friendly. You do not need footwear—you can exercise barefoot and if possible outdoors, which enhances body sensations.

Many exercises can be done at work or in the office, without having to change. However, if you exercise with the foam roller your clothes may wrinkle; therefore, choose suitable exercises when in the office. A thin exercise mat is also useful, but not essential.

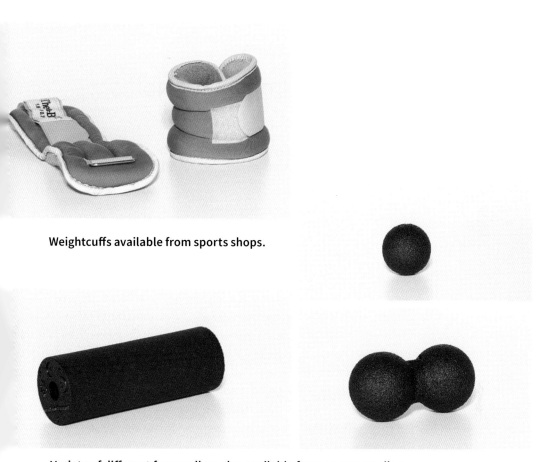

Weightcuffs available from sports shops.

Variety of different foam rollers also available from sports retailers.

Getting Started: Important Notes

● Take care if you are elderly or suffer from any disease. Although anyone can train their fascia, the elderly and chronically ill should exercise only after consultation with a medical professional.

● Children must be supervised: they should not practice on their own, and in particular not with a foam roller. The fascia training is not suitable for children under six years of age.

● Safety first: it is very important to warm up at the beginning! For all the springing-type exercises, or springs, you must be well warmed up and have good body awareness, as exercising when cold can lead to injury. When you put your exercises together, do not start with the elastic springs; begin instead with some warm-up exercises, in particular in the fields of feel and revive. This activates your receptors and identifies the limitations. Warm up well, and gradually increase the load.

● Less is more when you exercise the fascia: do not overload the tissue. Unlike muscle training, it is not necessary to go to the upper force limit when training the fascia. Design your own personal fascia program and perform it on a regular basis. Fascia changes slowly, but the gains will be long lasting. With regard to springs, a few repetitions with intervals is best: jump or swing only three to five times at the beginning, and then take a break of maybe one minute before you go to the next round. This way, you will allow the tissue time to recover.

● Practice consciously: always stay in a state of mindful perception when practicing and make sure that your movements feel smooth. Train your perception, do not become distracted when you practice, and do not watch television or conduct a lengthy conversation.

● Exercise regularly: you will notice visible signs of improvement after the first training session, but the more sustainable changes in architecture of your fascia will come after approximately three months. If you work out regularly twice a week, you become more flexible and agile. After two years, you can congratulate yourself on an entirely renewed fascial network in your body.

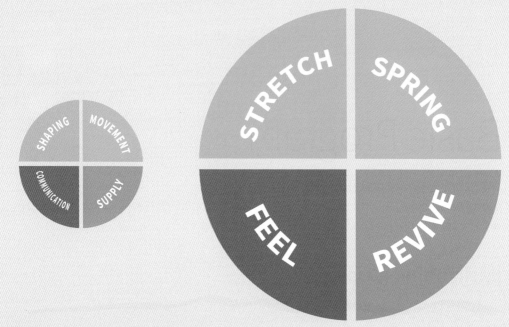

Your Guide:
The Four Dimensions of Fascia Training

You read about our four principles of training in the previous chapter. This circle with the four principles will guide you through each exercise. The area of the circle is highlighted in a certain color and indicates the origin of each exercise. This will help you to classify the exercises, and if you put a program together yourself, then you will be able to easily find appropriate exercises corresponding to the various segments of the circle. You should always cover all four principles in your individual training program.

The four training principles correspond to the four basic functions you have learned in Chapter 2 (p. 26):

TRAINING:
Stretch + Spring + Feel + Revive

FUNCTION:
Shaping + Movement + Communication + Supply

If you concentrate on all four principles of training, you will stimulate the four basic functions of your fascia—and thus provide optimum care and maintenance for your fascia network.

Basic Program

The basic program is an everyday training regime for everyone: it is suitable for beginners, sports newcomers, and inexperienced people. You can influence several important body-wide fascial chains with this compact series of exercises.

Basic Training Tips

● Train for about 10 minutes, once or twice a week—this is our recommended minimum program. You can of course train more often and longer: three to four times per week is good, depending on your needs. Make sure that exercises from the spring sector are performed for the same body part no more than twice a week, and that you then allow two or three days' rest between sessions. Exercises from other sectors can be performed more often. Even in a more intense program it is advisable to rest the fascial tissues for one day per week for optimal regeneration, without any targeted exercise stimulation.

● A few minutes of repetitions per exercise are enough—for example, in the morning before work. You can integrate these exercises into your existing fitness program at home or at work. The basic training program is well suited to warming up prior to a run or before sports activity.

● We start with warming up and proceed first with foot exercises, followed by the back, swing, and neck exercises.

● Always do the exercises of basic training in this order to warm your body up, as this will protect against strains and injuries.

OVERVIEW

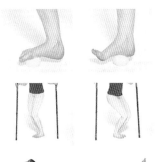

1. Rolling Out the Feet

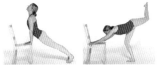

2. Calves and Achilles Tendon: Elastic Jumps

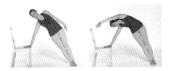

3. Front and Rear Line Stretches: Eagle Flight

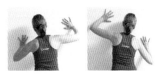

4. Waist and Side Stretches: Eagle Wings on a Chair

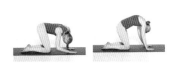

5. Shoulder and Shoulder Girdle Activation:
    Spring-Backs Against a Wall

6. Neck and Back Relaxation: Snake Dance

1. ROLLING OUT THE FEET

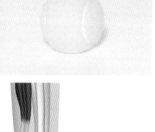

Maintains a healthy spring in the foot: the plantar fascia.

We start with an exercise from the revive sector. Using a tennis ball or similar, you roll out the large fascia under the feet, called the *plantar fascia*.

As you perform this procedure the plantar fascia is repeatedly squeezed out and filled with new fluid, and different movements and mechanical sensors are activated.

The plantar fascia runs under the foot from the heel to the ball of the toes, and is one of the thickest fascial tissues in the human body.

This thick plate, however, also needs to be flexible; if not, there can be adverse reactions, such as inflammation or heel spur pain, which are both very painful. Ideally, the heel pad should be able to move forward slightly in relation to the heel bone underneath, which will allow the Achilles tendon to transmit tension to the plantar fascia, and the other way round. Foot rolling with the ball promotes this mobility and stimulates this important fascial connection. The exercise can also have an effect right up to the back: after Rolling Out the Feet, many practitioners feel that after completing the self-treatment of one foot they can bend over more easily and can touch the ground more easily on this side, even with straight knees—try it out!

❶ Stand in bare feet, in a slightly stepped-forward position. Put a tennis ball or similar under the front foot, directly behind the toes.

❷ Now gradually transfer more and more weight from your rear foot onto the front foot, and thus onto the ball. Slowly increase the weight on the front foot as long as it feels comfortable. You may possibly feel a pleasant well-being pain—a feeling of pleasant pressure. This is expected, and indicates the spot where the fascia is stuck together. Stay here a moment longer and roll into this spot with small movements.

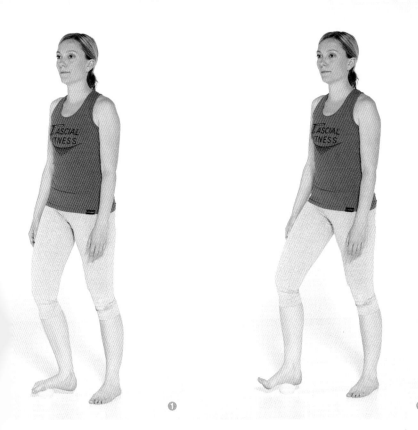

① ②

❸ – ❺   Next move the foot forward, so that the ball rolls very slowly, as if in slow motion, from the toes toward the heel, while applying steady pressure. Let the ball become almost immersed in your foot, and experiment with different angles and directions. In this way, you will stimulate the entire sole of the foot.

Do this exercise for approximately two minutes, first with one foot, then with the other.

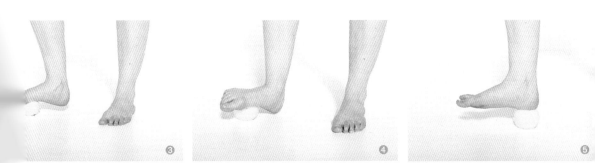

③ ④ ⑤

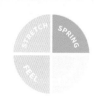

2. CALVES AND ACHILLES TENDON: ELASTIC JUMPS

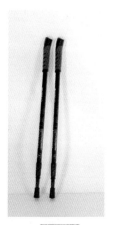

These small, flexible jumps are performed using sticks for support, but can also be effective without support. If you want to work with sticks, we recommend standard Nordic walking sticks or similar poles.

Elastic Jumps specifically train the Achilles tendon, or heel cord; this is the most important fibrous tissue band for walking and running and has to be tear resistant and stretchy. If the tendon is poorly trained and its supply is inadequate, ensuing problems may lead to Achilles tendon injury.

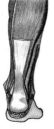

Achilles tendon and calf aponeurosis.

The calf aponeurosis also plays an important role in walking and running: this is the upward extension of the Achilles tendon and reaches upwards to just below the knee.

Shortening of the Achilles tendon and calf aponeurosis are probably the reason that Western adults often cannot squat like they did as a child. In other cultures, this is frequently different, where squatting and sitting is part of the daily routine—as a result, even in adulthood, the tendon remains well stretched.

You will not feel a change in the tendon overnight by exercising it: the time required for the transformation of fascia is several months. It is also beneficial to spring about or to walk barefoot more often; each instance of hopping, jumping, and jogging or running barefoot can support the transformation of the fascia in the feet and calves. Remember, however, to allow sufficient adaptation time – and to increase the load in many small steps over several months – when applying non-habitual loading challenges to your connective tissues, as they can take a long time to adapt.

To prepare yourself, take a few steps in bare feet and apply significant pressure with your heel into the floor. Then, with increasing speed, start to rock the heels on the ground; be aware of the impact pressure of the heels against the ground. Now the actual exercise starts.

❶ – ❷ Rest on the sticks and hop slightly upward: this should be done as lightly as possible. Avoid the heel thumping down and do not slam the foot flat on the floor. The less sound you hear from your feet, the better the exercise!

If you find a sense of ease when you jump, just like a rubber ball, then your fascia is active. Perform just three to five repetitions and then take a short break. Keep your heels on the ground or take a few steps on the floor before you start the next round. This is important so that the tissue can recover between the sets of jumps; moreover, through this movement the fluid can be pressed out and then flow back to the fascia again.

❸ – ❹ Variation: Jump laterally back and forth, or jump in a twisting motion by turning your toes inward and outward. If you are inexperienced, you can omit the sticks. Always make sure to jump as silently as possible. With time you will feel that you can consciously control and catch your weight on the toes and front of the foot.

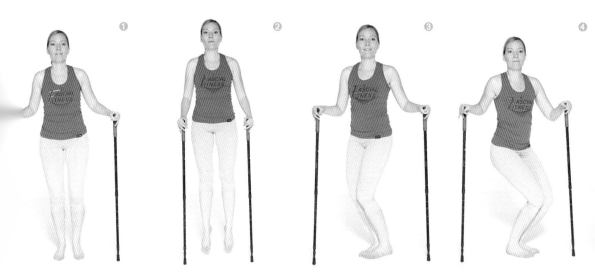

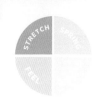

3. FRONT AND REAR LINE STRETCHES: EAGLE FLIGHT

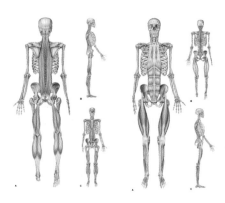

**Eagle flight
– back line.**

**Eagle flight
– front line.**

This exercise stretches the connective tissue in the posterior thigh at the hip. It stimulates the front and back long fascia chains.

People who spend a lot of time in a seated position often have shortened fascia along the back line up the legs. There is a simple test for this: lean forward while standing. Can you touch the ground with your fingertips without bending your knees? If not, then the fascia at the back of your thighs is probably shortened. The connective tissue is connected from the thigh up to the sacrum, then all the way into the back; the lower back is therefore affected by reduced mobility. This can cause back pain and a resulting decrease in mobility of the hip joints.

❶ Stand in front of a solid chair, keeping your legs about hip-width apart. Step back about 1 m and put both hands in a straight position on the seat of the chair. Your weight should be mainly on your feet, with your hands only lightly touching the seat.

❷ Now push down against the seat with your hands and slightly bend one knee. Push your weight through your hands onto the chair.

❸ Do the same with the other knee slightly bent.

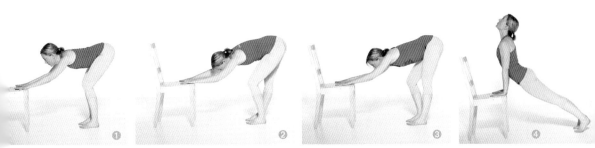

4 Next put all your weight onto your hands and straighten your back with your head up high.

5 – 6 Push up your back and stand on tiptoe. Come back down to the starting position.

7 – 8 Now lift one leg up and back in a straight line with your body. Repeat with the other leg. Try varying the stretching movements: push your back all the way rearward, make a high arch, then lift one leg up; bend and stretch in various positions.

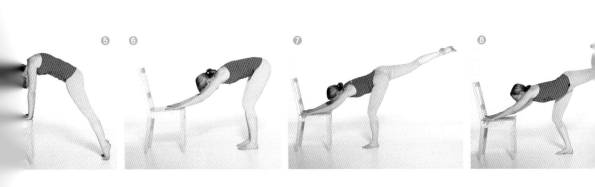

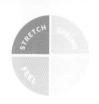

4. WAIST AND SIDE STRETCHES: EAGLE WINGS ON A CHAIR

Hips, thighs, and body core are often underused through sitting down for long periods, but unfortunately many people in everyday life stay in a seated position for too long. With the following exercise, you will stretch these structures and call into play the side fascial chains, the lateral lines, which stabilize the body.

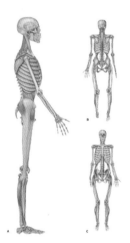

The lateral lines stabilize the body.

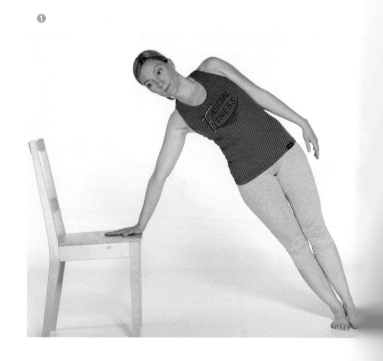

❶ Put a stable stool or a chair close to the wall so that it cannot slip away. With one hand, rest laterally in a tilted position with both legs extended.

❷ Bring the whole body into a long stretch, and make sure that your lower side is not sagging—it should remain straight and stretched. Then lift your free arm over your head in an arch, and stretch the side of your body.

❸ – ❹ You can vary the position of the hand and try the stretches with different angles and directions of the upper arm; you can also experiment with your own variations.

Always make sure that your body is not sagging toward the floor: correct your posture if necessary. Rise up slowly until you reach a standing position, and repeat the exercise on the other side. Perform this exercise ten times on each side.

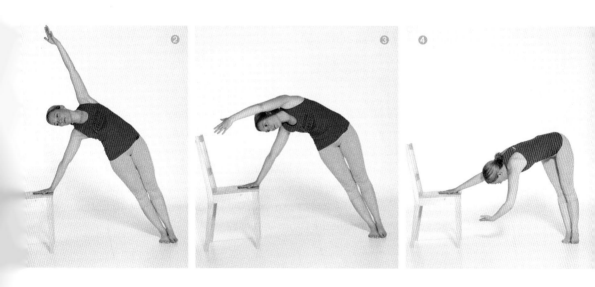

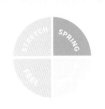

5. SHOULDERS AND SHOULDER GIRDLE ACTIVATION: SPRING -BACKS AGAINST A WALL

Those of us who sit at a desk for long periods often suffer shoulder problems; this occurs because of the long-term stationary position, which our bodies are not specifically designed for. The shoulder area contains very firm, thick fascia which connects at the front to the pectoral muscle.

The system links the back and the arms at the front downward to the waist. As we evolved, our original design allowed us to swing from tree to tree; however, sitting for long periods, especially in the unnatural position at a desk, leads to tension in many areas of the body. Parts of fascia in the shoulder joint can become stiff and painful, which can be quite stressful and can also lead to what is known as *frozen shoulder*.

A flexible, well-trained shoulder area is less prone to stiffness—the following simple exercise can be carried out on a wall at home or at the office. It is quite versatile, because it trains the abdomen, shoulder, and back all at the same time. This exercise activates the structures in the shoulder girdle.

❶ – ❷ Stand in front of a wall at a distance of 0.5 to 1 m. Begin relatively close to the wall, and then increase the distance as you progress. You will be tipping forward to bring your weight onto the hands, but before you begin, rub your palms together vigorously a few times, so that you warm up the perception in your hands. Then place your palms on the wall and feel the contact with the wall for a moment; next, push away from the wall, relax, and let yourself go back toward the wall. Push yourself off dynamically with both hands again. The action is similar to upright press-ups against a wall.

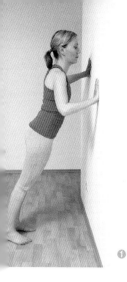 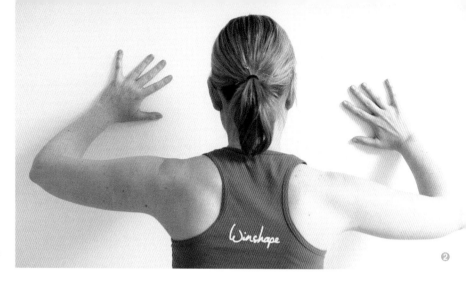

The spring-back should be easy and effortless, as if the wall is a trampoline. If it feels like a chore, then you are working the muscles too hard. In this case, try to use the springiness of your fascia—move closer to the wall and try to find the dynamic, effortless fascia rhythms.

❸ – ❹ Pull the lower abdomen slightly inward to stabilize the midsection and also to avoid a hollow back. Try some variations: place your hands diagonally to the left, and sometimes to the right. Repeat six or seven times.

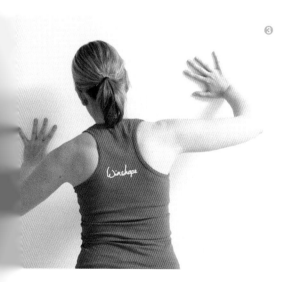 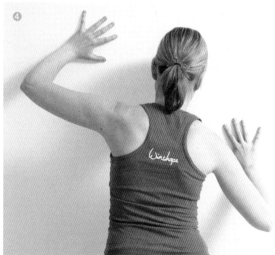

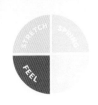

6. NECK AND BACK RELAXATION: SNAKE DANCE

Neck pain frequently occurs in combination with a headache. That is no coincidence: the neck fascia runs from behind and over the head to the eyebrows. A little further down the neck, around the shoulders, the fascia is very soft. The neck has to be very flexible so that you have sufficient mobility to turn your head easily. It is therefore important to both preserve the mobility of the neck fascia and consolidate it. In all the exercises around the neck you should proceed very gently and slowly.

❶   Kneel on the floor or on a mat, with the knees about hip-width apart and the arms shoulder-width apart. Begin to undulate slowly with snakelike movements in a wave along your spine.

❷   Start by lifting the sternum and arching your back, and then let the sternum fall slowly toward the ground. Keep the lumbar spine under control and stretch the tailbone. The movement should be fluid and feel quite pleasant.

❸ – ❺   Now try lateral oscillations: move in larger sideways movements between the shoulders, back and forth, then finally in a figure of eight and circular movements.

❻ – ❽   Experiment with different directions and wave movements. Do the complete exercise for a few minutes. At the end, make the movements smaller and finer, then slowly straighten up and relax for a few moments.

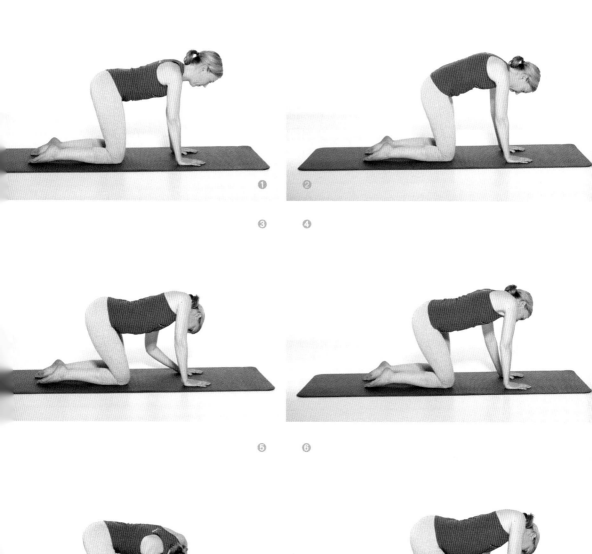

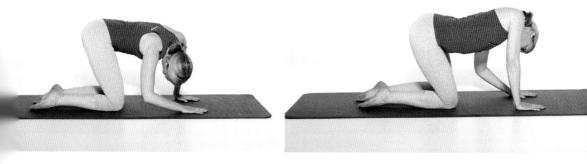

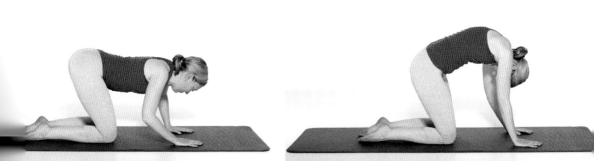

Exercises for Problem Areas: Back, Neck, Arms, Hips, Feet

The following series of exercises covers individual problem areas or issues from specific angles. Always think about the entire network of your fascia, and work out holistically. Integrate this small series, or selected exercises, into your regular basic training program.

PROGRAMS FOR PROBLEM AREAS

1. **Short Back Program**

2. **At the Office: Problems in the Neck, Arms, and Shoulders**

3. **Around the Hips**

4. **For the Feet and Stance**

A. SHORT BACK PROGRAM

Here is a mini workout for the back—five exercises, specifically aimed at the lumbar fascia, and covering all four training dimensions. It specifically protects against back pain but is also good for all those people who sit or stand for long periods. You can do these exercises two or three times a week, or add them to your usual workout. At least for the first few times, it is recommended to follow this order:

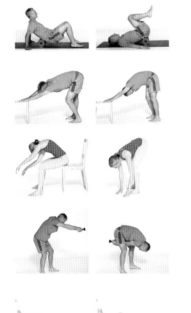

1. Rolling Out the Lumbar Fascia

2. Back Stretch: The Cat

3. African Bends

4. Flying Sword

5. Vertebral Chain Relief

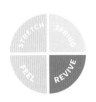

1. ROLLING OUT THE LUMBAR FASCIA

We start with Rolling Out the Lumbar Fascia, which stimulates the tissue and ensures liquid exchange, so that the fascia can regenerate and repair damage. Here the fascia roll comes into play (see p. 107). If you want to do back exercises more often, then a fascia roll is really worthwhile; in the case of thigh and calf exercises, we always work with a fascia roll.

❶ Sit comfortably on the floor on a mat and push your upper body upwards from your arms. Then lift up your pelvis and place the fascia roll under your lumbar region.

❷ Roll a little toward the chest and then back again, with your arms crossed behind your head.

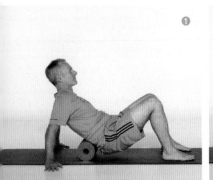
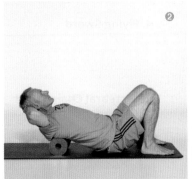
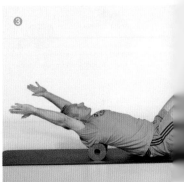

❸ Next stretch out your arms to open up your shoulder girdle. Roll slowly upward and downward.

❹ Now lift your legs in the air with the fascia roll against your lower back. Do this consciously and slowly.

❺ – ❻ Spread your hands laterally on the floor. Make sure that your back is becoming rounder and that the roll is below the hollow of your back. Now, in slow motion, begin to vary your position on the roll by small angles: change the position of the roll again and roll your entire back fascia.

Try to control the pressure, so that the experience feels like a back massage! No acute or sharp sensations should occur.

If lying down is difficult, you can do the exercise standing up against a wall, with support from your legs. You might be able to control the pressure more easily in this position.

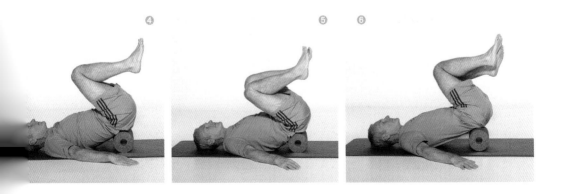

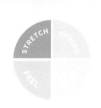

2. BACK STRETCH: THE CAT

In this exercise you will reach the superficial layer of the lumbar fascia; then, with the back straight, you repeat the exercise to treat the deeper layer.

❶ Take a chair and place it with the backrest against a wall. Step a few feet back and place both hands straight on the seat. Your weight rests mainly on your feet, with the hands placed lightly on the seat.

Stand with your feet about hip-width apart, with your arms extended and your hip joints positioned above the heels. Bend your knees slowly forward and simultaneously press your tailbone back and up like a cat, extending while stretching your buttocks upward.

❶

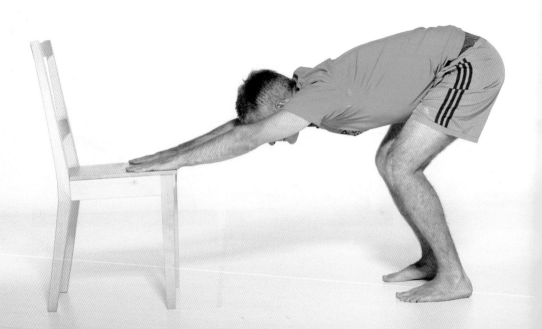

❷ Now let the right buttock rise up and backward: your right knee extends and your weight shifts to the left foot. Spread your right hand and slide the fingers forward on the chair seat. You should feel an intense stretch on your right side.

❸ Relax and repeat the exercise—right side, followed by the left.

Make sure to pull the lower abdomen actively inward; otherwise, the weight of the abdominal organs causes the lumbar spine to droop inward and a hollow back will occur. If you like a bit more of a challenge, then you can try this exercise while standing up without the chair.

❷   ❸

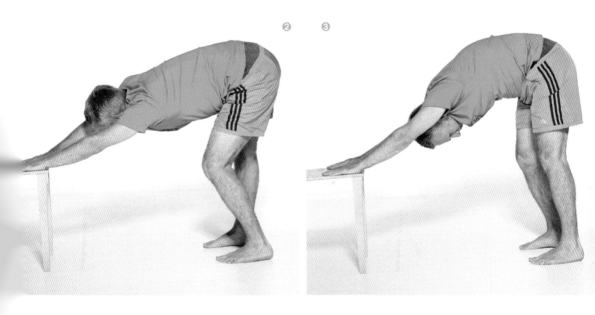

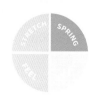

3. AFRICAN BENDS

The lumbar fascia not only distributes forces and holds muscles in place, but also acts as a mechanical control for human stance; we should therefore try to increase the elasticity of the lumbar fascia to combat back pain. This bending exercise is based on movements that researchers have observed in some regions of Africa. African people do similar springing movements in their backs while working in their fields. Though they are bent over, this is a remarkably natural and gentle posture that uses the storage power of the fascia.

❶ Sit upright on the front edge of a stable chair and open your legs slightly more than hip width.

❷ Lower your chin onto your chest and slowly roll your head downward until your fingertips touch the ground. Your knees should remain aligned above the toes.

❸ – ❹ Now try to pull yourself a tiny bit further down toward the floor. The fascia may tense as you try to go forward. Now let go and your lumbar fascia will spring back.

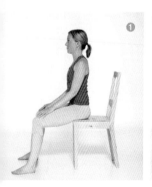 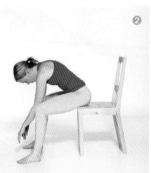 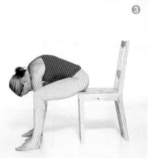 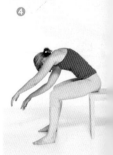

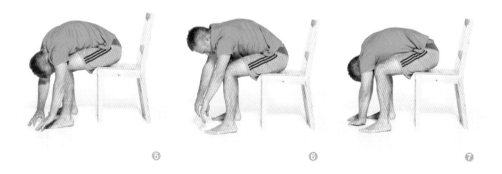

⑤ – ⑦   Find a rhythm that suits you, so that the movement does not put you under any strain. You should feel a resilient rubber-ball feeling in the lower back. Repeat this action with small changes in the angle of your arms and lower back, for five or six repetitions.

⑧ – ⑩   **Variation:** If you feel confident, this exercise can be done standing up. The knees should not be locked, but slightly bent.

With some people, the back will be naturally maintained fairly straight in such exercises, but for others it will be rounder—it just depends on the individual's mobility.

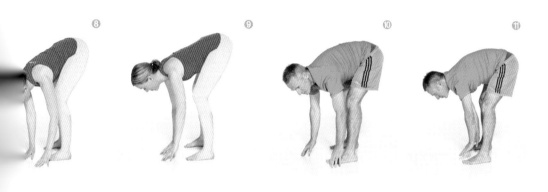

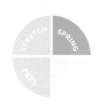

4. FLYING SWORD

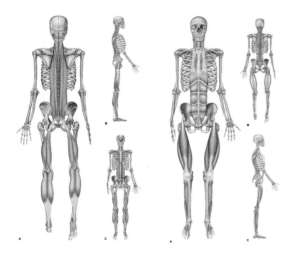

The superficial back line.

The superficial front line.

This exercise targets the lumbar fascia and the long fascia line of the front and back lines; these are important for the strength and stability of the spine.

The Flying Sword is very energizing and lively. However, note that this exercise should only be done when you are warmed up; moreover, if you suffer from back pain or spinal instability issues, you should begin gently. First try one or two gentle repetitions, so that you can detect whether this exercise has a stabilizing or destabilizing effect on your lower back because of your personal body structure. In the case of the latter, or if you are unsure, do not do this exercise.

❶ Hold one small 1.5 kg dumbbell (or as a substitute a small, filled water bottle) in both hands. Raise the dumbbell in an arching motion, upward and backward over the head.

Next start to move your upper body forward and backward, in slow snakelike movements; this brings into play the body's fascia and generates the momentum. The snakelike movements will pass through the stomach and chest, and there should be movement of the thoracic spine. Do five or six repetitions of these movements, while holding the dumbbell behind your head.

❷ – ❹ Now look up and forward from the sternum. Bring your upper body down and swing your arms with the dumbbell passing backward between your legs and then back up over your head. Straighten your arms naturally into the swing. Do this smoothly and gently.

Swing six or seven times, from top to bottom and back again. Then, at the same time as you swing up, move to the left and to the right. Try at least 20 repetitions, but make sure you are not putting too much strain on your lower back, as it can become overloaded.

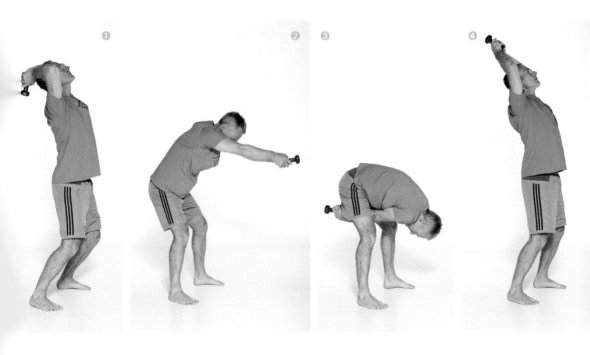

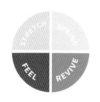

5. VERTEBRAL CHAIN RELIEF

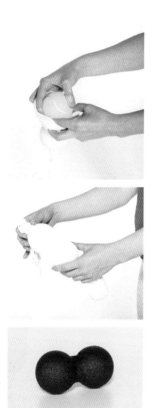

The spine is like a chain of moving links, and thanks to the fascial tension system, the back remains stable and upright (covered in Chapter 2). We call the spine, the vertebral chain, and try to restore its mobility using this exercise, whereby the fascial structures in the postural muscles of the *vertebral chain* are stimulated and relaxed.

For this exercise you will need two tennis balls wrapped in a knotted sock or stocking. Alternatively, a double ball which is specifically designed for such exercises can be purchased from a sports shop.

❶ Lie flat on the floor in front of a chair, with your legs on the seat. You can place a blanket under your pelvis or calves for comfort. Hold the sock containing the tennis balls in your hand.

❷ First loosen the back generally as you consciously begin to connect your sacrum, which is the lowest part of your back, with the ground. Make small tentative movements toward the floor with the lower part of your back. Then slowly lift your whole vertebral chain off the ground and move one vertebra at a time back to the ground. Repeat this three times.

❸   Now lift up your lower back and push the sock with the tennis balls under the thoracic spine, so that the balls are placed either side of the vertebral column. The spinous processes will then have enough space because of this gap between the balls in the middle. Only continue if you feel that the balls are contacting muscle and not bone.

❹ – ❻   Now slowly bring your weight down onto the balls and increase the pressure. Again you can make small angle changes to the contact points with the balls. Stay in this position as long as you find it comfortable. Then move the balls further down the back, one vertebra at a time, and repeat the exercise.

By doing this exercise you will work down to the sacrum step by step. At this point, remove the balls and feel contact with the floor for a moment. Do you notice a change?

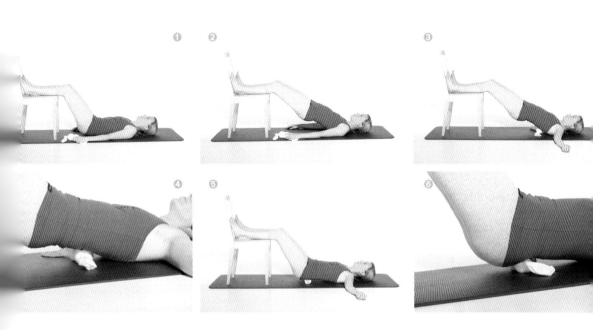

B. AT THE OFFICE: PROBLEMS IN THE NECK, ARMS, AND SHOULDERS

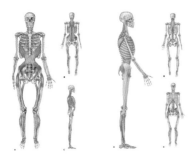

Exercises for those who work in offices or at a desk:

The fascia of the spinal and lateral lines is not utilized efficiently when sitting continuously. One often spends almost the entire day in a long-term seated position. When working at a desk, or looking at a computer screen, the arms rest mostly in an unfavorable position on the desk. Shoulder–neck–arm syndromes are common issues arising from permanent sitting positions, even more so than deep lower back pain. The exercises below relieve the overburdened fascia in this area. Additionally, they encourage the long fascia lines which run through the legs, arms, and torso, particularly those mentioned in Chapter 3—the lateral and spiral lines, which waste away when sitting continuously.

These exercises can be done at home or at the office, or they can enhance your regular fascia program twice a week. The swinging exercise (Swinging Bamboo, p. 142) should only be done after the body has been warmed up. The Spring-Backs Against a Wall is the same as that in the basic program (p. 122), and can be integrated at the end of this series.

1. Shoulder Stretch

2. Freedom for the Neck

3. Relaxation for Tired Forearms

4. Momentum for the Whole Body (Swinging Bamboo)

SHOULDER STRETCH

In this exercise try to identify the points at which the angular momentum for you is particularly noticeable.

❶ Stand by a door frame, wall, or cabinet, as shown in the image. Place your hand flat on the surface, then move a little forward and stretch the arm and shoulder.

❷ – ❸ You can experiment with small angle changes to activate the different fibers. Furthermore, change the position of your hand—place it higher and lower; change the angle of your body to the wall too, in order to vary the stretch.

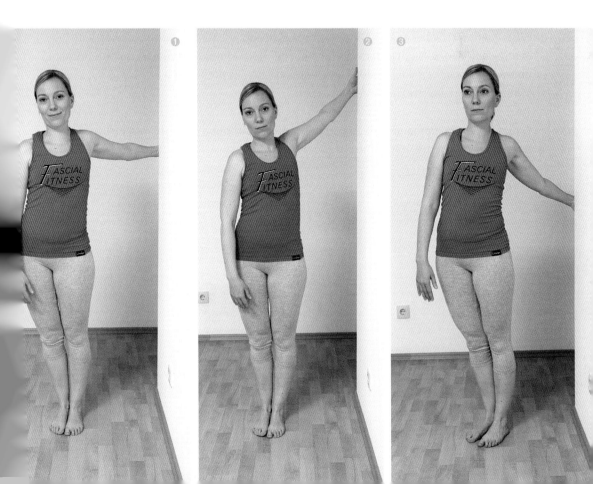

FREEDOM FOR THE NECK

This exercise relieves the cervical spine and all the fascial elements around the neck, shoulders, and head. Only rarely do we sit so precisely aligned that the weight of the head floats just above the vortex chain, which would be the ideal situation. As a result, the muscles need to do a lot of balancing work, which can cause the entire shoulder area to become tense and the cervical spine to be overloaded. With this exercise you can loosen this particular area of your neck.

❶ You will need an inflated balloon for this exercise. Place yourself in front of a chair, with your legs hip-width apart, and hold the balloon in your hands. Tighten your abdomen a little and roll, vertebra by vertebra, down to the seat of the chair. Place the balloon on the seat and put the top of your head on the balloon. Your hands support you loosely on the seat.

Experiment with small angle changes in the neck, and roll gently into the balloon with just your head, moving slightly back and forth. Your neck should be very loose and relaxed. Control the weight of your head on the balloon—do not press too hard. Try to make your movements smaller and more varied.

❷ It is even more demanding if you do this exercise without a balloon, with just your head placed directly on the seat of the chair.

❶   ❷

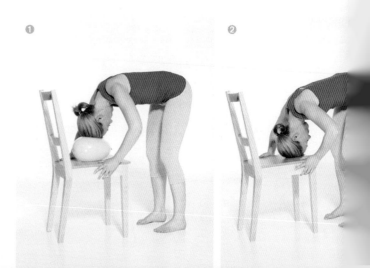

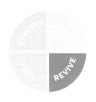

RELAXATION FOR TIRED FOREARMS

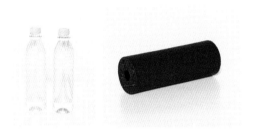

This exercise is ideal for breaks in the office routine, when your forearms are suffering from long periods in the same position. You will need a small filled water bottle or a small fascia roll (see images, A Blackroll mini-roll 15 cm long, 5.4 cm thick).

❶ Place the water bottle or the fascia roll in front of you on the table, desk, or chair, and rest your forearm on it.

❷ – ❸ Put just your arm weight onto the bottle or roll, and relax. Starting slowly, in millimeter-size movements, roll out your forearm. Work up to rolling the length of the arm, from your elbow to your hand, and vice versa. Adjust the rolling action by making many small angle changes.

Proceed in slow motion and imagine that you are pressing out water from a sponge with this movement.

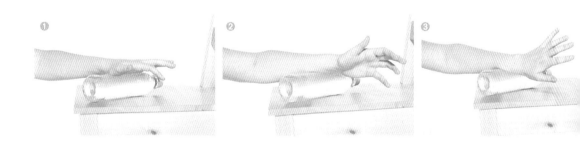

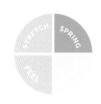

MOMENTUM FOR THE WHOLE BODY: SWINGING BAMBOO

For this exercise you will need a small dumbbell, about 0.5 to 1.5 kg in weight. As a substitute you can use a small filled water bottle.

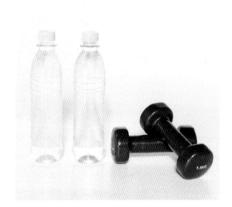

❶ – ❷ Stand in a stable position, like a sumo wrestler. We call this position *prior force*: the legs should be slightly wider than the hips, the toes should point slightly outward, and the knees should be slightly bent over the toes. Keep your back straight and imagine that you are pulling a small weight down at your coccyx. Holding the dumbbell with both hands in front of your body, swing it in small circles to encourage rotation of the vertebral chain: this slowly warms up the structures. Perform these circle swings for about a minute.

❶
❷

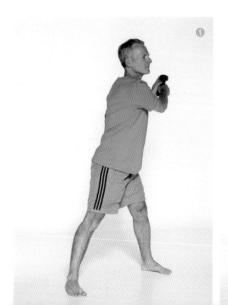

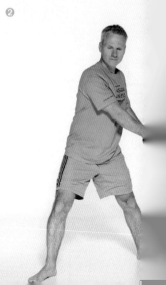

❸ Now swing for a few repetitions on one side, diagonally upward and backward, moving the legs at the same time. Bend your knees to the same side as your swing, and stretch the other leg out. Open your arms while swinging. When you swing to the right, let go of the dumbbell (or bottle) with your left hand. Swing with your right arm, together with the dumbbell in the hand, diagonally upward to the right, and rotate the torso up to the right. This gives power to the long fascia, specifically the spiral line. Note that the outer edge of the left foot remains firmly anchored on the ground; conversely, as you do the exercise to the left side, the right foot stays put.

❹ – ❻   Remain in this position for a moment, and maintain the stability of the outside of the foot of your extended leg, up to the hand with the dumbbell, by doing small springs. Then look up and back down again: your whole side should be tense. Swing from the chest diagonally back down; this movement should follow a smooth curve and not be overextended. Be aware of your body's signals: if you feel that you have understood the physics of the movement, then you can perform three to five repetitions in the upper position without a break. Relax, then switch to the other side.

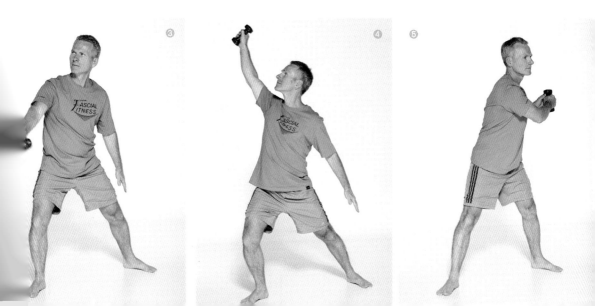

C. AROUND THE HIPS

Because pain and loss of motion at the hip joint are very common, this small set of exercises for the hips will appeal to many people.

Hip surgery is unfortunately one of the most frequent operations in the Western world. After the knee, the hip is the next largest joint in the human body; it contains the strongest ligaments of the entire body. It is therefore no wonder that the state of the fascial elements of the hip play such a large role in movement. In each step we take, the hip joints and ligaments are used, and this joint must be extremely mobile. Continuous sitting causes mechanically detrimental stretching, and at the same time underuses the joint, which affects the nutrition of the cartilage in the joint. Certain sports, such as cycling, are not optimal for the supply and mobility of the hip, and we should therefore compensate for this with appropriate exercises (see p. 180).

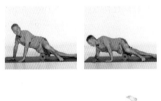

1. Rolling out the Thigh

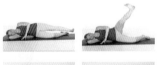

2. Activating the Outer Thigh

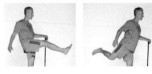

3. Swinging the Legs

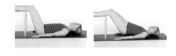

4. The Skate

ROLLING OUT THE THIGH

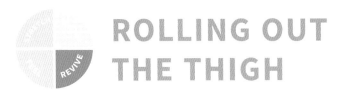

For this exercise you will need a fascia roll.

❶ Assume the start position by lying on your right side, with your weight on the right hand, so that your elbow is below the right armpit. Place the foam roll just below the femoral head (lower hip). Stretch your lower leg and pull the upper leg up and over the right leg. Support your upper body with your free left hand.

❷ Now slowly roll down from the outside of the top of the thigh (trochanter) toward the knee. As you press slowly over the roll, imagine your thigh is a sponge. If you find areas that are particularly tight or painful, hold the position for half a minute to a minute, and relax slowly into the pressure while making tiny angle changes. Make sure to keep your head in line with your spine. You can also do the exercise with your right arm bent and the forearm supported on the ground, taking the weight of the upper body.

❸ When the roll reaches a point just above the knee, slowly roll back up to the trochanter. After the second pass, you may already feel a soothing "dissolving" in the tissue. Finally, remove the roll and feel the release in your inner thigh.

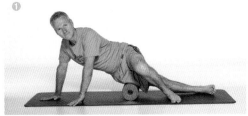

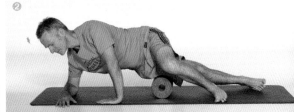

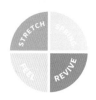

ACTIVATING THE OUTER THIGH

❶ Lie down on your side on the floor. The bottom leg should be slightly bent, with the upper leg floating in a slightly raised position above the ground. Be sure to stretch the back and to not allow the spine to sag sideways (down).

❷ Next, bend the knee and slide the foot out from the leg in front of the body, as if you wanted to push away an imaginary wall.

❶
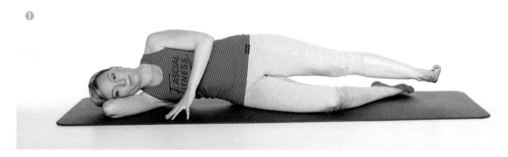

❷
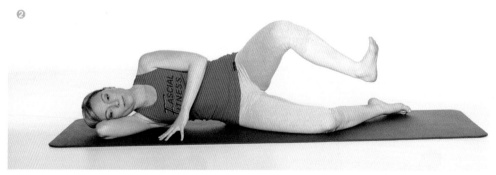

❸
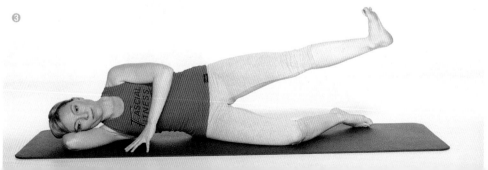

❸ When you reach full knee extension, stretch a bit further out at the heel and then on each individual toe. Make sure that you remain in the side position. Bend the knee slightly and slide your leg out again like a telescope, this time by extending the lumbar chain down and out.

❹ – ❺ Adjust the motion by making small rotational changes and using various angles; slide the leg in different directions—upward, forward, and diagonally.

To change sides, slowly curl up with your knees drawn to your chest and roll over onto the other side.

❻ – ❼ If you are looking for a bigger challenge, instead of lying down on the ground you can position yourself sideways on a chair, or you could put on weight cuffs. However, always make sure that you have enough stability in the trunk and cervical chain, so as not to overload these structures.

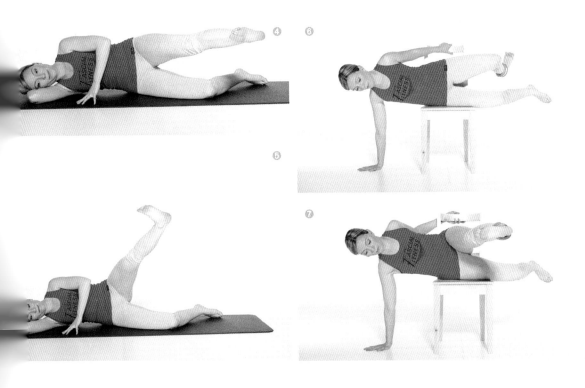

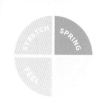

SWINGING THE LEGS

Use a Nordic walking stick and low stool. This exercise can be done in bare feet.

❶ Stand on a low stool, and take one of your Nordic walking poles for support. Start on the left-hand side and lean with your left hand onto the pole, keeping the right hand free. The left foot stands securely on the stool, with the knee slightly bent, and your right foot should be loose by the stool. Now begin to swing lightly with the right leg. The swings should be slow and controlled, so that the leg moves back and forth like a pendulum.

❷ – ❸ Next, concentrate on fascial momentum: move your free leg back carefully and stretch the front connective tissue, and then bring the leg forward quickly from the pelvis. Be careful not to stretch the muscles above the leg too much, to ensure that the spring mechanism of the fascia is working.

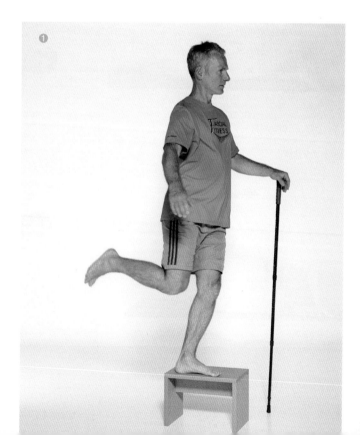

Swing the entire leg back and forth smoothly in a rhythmic motion. Feel your hip and the whole side of the upper body to the right, and in front over the chest to the left arm. You can increase the rebound effect by making sure that the momentum of the leg swing results from the pulling back of your pubic bone.

Change sides after about three minutes.

More experienced people can perform this exercise without a stick; it can also be practiced on a step. When you feel comfortable you could do the exercise simply on the ground: stand straight up with your legs hip-width apart, then shift your weight onto one leg and swing the other. In the beginning, to maintain your balance hold with one hand onto a windowsill or a chair. After a while, also try this exercise without support, so that you can concentrate on the swing of the free leg.

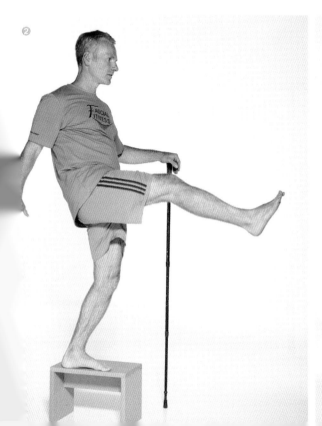
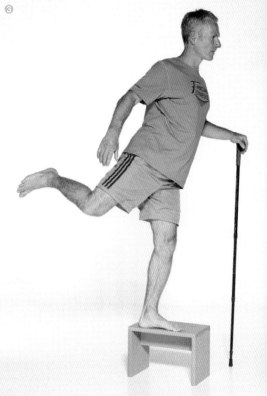

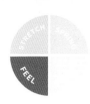

THE SKATE

① Lie flat in front of a stable chair and position your lower legs parallel on the seat. Place your sacrum (the lowest part of your pelvis) on the floor. Try different contact points and angle changes.

② Next, slowly lift up your pelvis by extending your tailbone. Now use different curves, spirals, and waves with your raised pelvis—like a skate that floats through the sea.

Proceed slowly and deliberately, and be aware of your inner impulses for the next move.

Finally, let your pelvis sink gently down, vertebra by vertebra, to the floor, before launching into the next round. Repeat three times.

①   ②

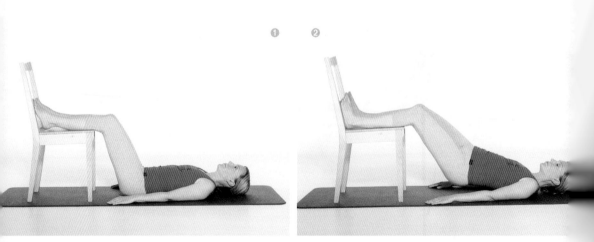

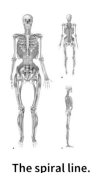

The spiral line.

D. FOR THE FEET AND STANCE

Thanks to the catapult effect of the muscles and tendons, walking is the most energy-efficient mode of transport for people. How well this works depends on the body's awareness and balance, and on the elastic storage capability of the fascia. The transitions in walking are reproduced along the fascial chains, which we covered in Chapter 2, and these therefore play an important role. The spiral line is responsible for balance and tracking when walking.

The following short series of exercises shows you how to practice several important functions relating to the feet and posture.

People who walk a lot, and also those who spend a significant amount of time sitting, should regularly stretch their Achilles tendon. Others who spend lengthy periods on their feet can create a lot of energy by regularly strengthening the fascia in the feet and lower legs with elastic jumping. We begin and end this series with exercises for vitality and awareness.

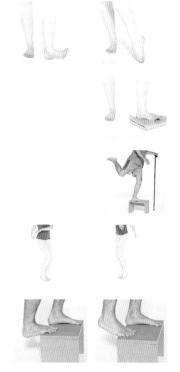

1. Rolling out the Plantar Fascia

2. Sensitizing the Soles of the Feet

3. Swinging the Legs

4. Elastic Jumping for the Feet, Calves, and Achilles Tendon

5. Stretching the Achilles Tendon

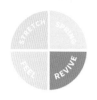

ROLLING OUT THE PLANTAR FASCIA

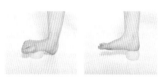

Begin by rolling out the plantar fascia as in the first exercise of the basic program (see p. 114). Put particular emphasis on the heel pad.

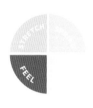

SENSITIZING THE SOLES OF THE FEET

❶ – ❻ Stand with your legs hip-width apart. Shift your weight to one side and begin to feel the floor with the other foot in small micro-movements.

Adjust the amount of pressure on the floor, and slide various contact points of your foot into the ground. Proceed slowly and work your way over the entire sole of the foot.

Next, take a moment to relax on both legs. Have you noticed the difference? The exercise can even have a relaxing effect on the entire body. Repeat the exercise on the other side.

❼ Try this exercise on different surfaces—carpet, tile, wood, or mat—or with a towel under the foot. Consciously note the differences.

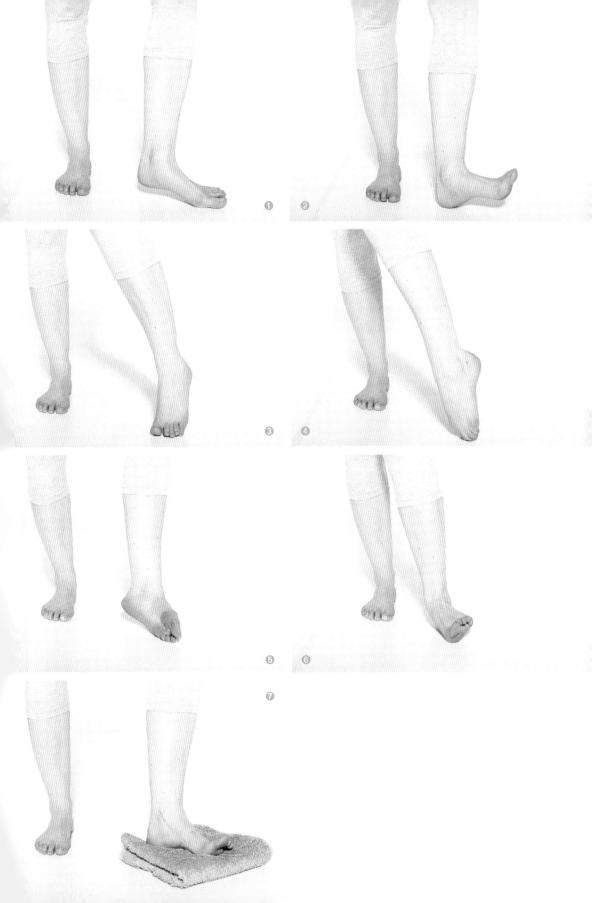

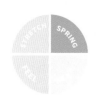

SWINGING THE LEGS

This exercise was described in the series for the hips on p. 148. The hip movement that you practice can even be used while walking. We know from hiking or walking with others that sometimes we go too fast or beyond our own natural pace, and so we need more energy. In short, we are not walking with optimal efficiency—or "fascially," as we say. Try to bend the rear leg in small walking movements, as learned in the swinging exercise; relax before you take your next step forward, and go at your own pace. With this exercise, you will improve the use of your fascia and save muscle energy.

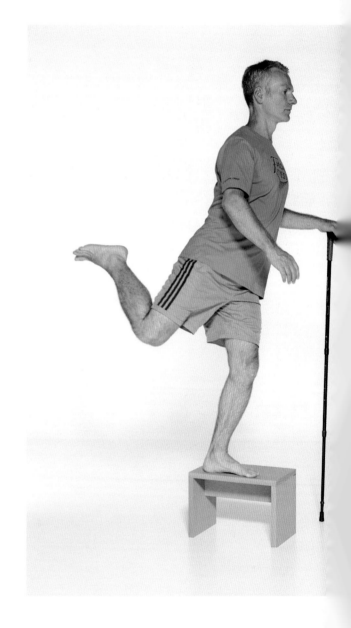

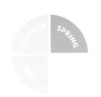
ELASTIC JUMPING FOR THE FEET, CALVES, AND ACHILLES TENDON

The next exercise is the short series that has already been covered in the basic program under Elastic Jumps on p. 116.

These jumps train particularly the Achilles tendon and all the muscles and fascia in the feet and lower legs. This exercise can be performed with or without poles, and is best done barefoot.

It is important to keep a smooth and energy-efficient transition; moreover, as already mentioned, you should include a variety of typical movements from everyday life—walking, hopping, jumping, and dancing—and do the exercise barefoot.

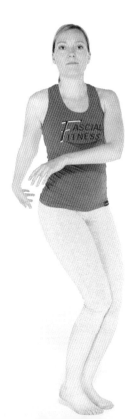
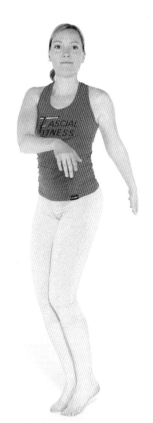

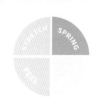

STRETCHING THE ACHILLES TENDON

We already know how important the state of the Achilles tendon is, as we covered this topic earlier, in the exercises for the basic program (see p. 116). Stretching the Achilles tendon is particularly important for those who run regularly and spend long periods standing up— but even more so for older people, for Viking types with stiff tissues, and for athletes.

❶ Stand on a stool. Pull back one heel a little and let it float freely, while keeping the other foot flat on the stool.

❷ – ❸ Now push the floating heel down and hold this position for a few moments. Then vary the position of the heel using small angle changes to achieve a stretch in the various fibers.

Take care not to overstretch, and decide when you need to rest for a while. Maintain the whole body erect and tense. You can also stretch your arms up above the head in order to involve the whole body. Instead of a stool, you could use a stair step for this exercise.

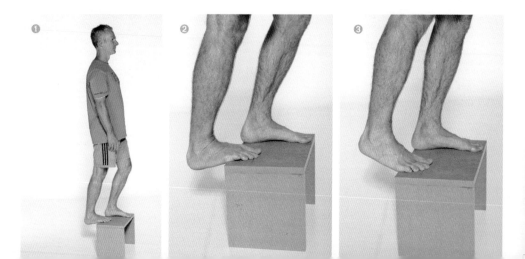

Tips and Exercises for Flexible People and Vikings

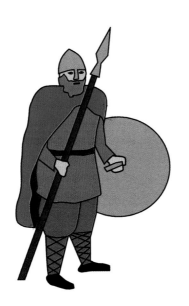
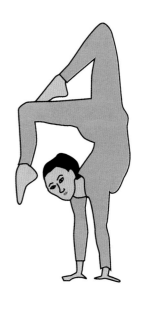

This section presents some important information and exercises that are particularly useful for the various types of connective tissue, especially the ones at either end of the scale in the image below.

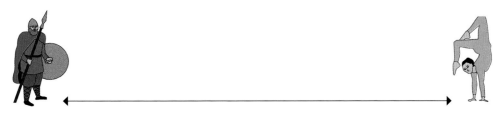

Spectrum of normal types.

FLEXIBLE PEOPLE WITH SOFT CONNECTIVE TISSUE

■ Stretch

It is not advisable to stretch too far and too hard: keep the range of your stretching exercises small and controlled. Learn how to make small, deliberate changes in the stretch positions to train your body awareness of the joints. For energetic people, the objective is not to become more flexible, or increase the range of motion, but rather to develop an awareness of the joints and tissue and of what the limits are. We should avoid straining in the extreme ranges of the joints.

■ Spring

Take care when you spring. Perform your springing exercises strongly and actively, but do not work under too much strain. You should spring in a position in which the muscles you are working are not intensely stretched. Recognize the fact that the desired position is when these muscles are shortened and thickened to the greatest extent: only in this state do the tissues become firmer through short and springy stretches.

■ Revive

The revive sector includes some hearty, jolting, quick mini-rolling movements that are beneficial, as they stimulate the connective tissue to increase collagen production.

■ Feel

Exercises from the feel sector are particularly important for you. It is common with gymnastic types for the self-examination to be inaccurate when they attempt extreme stretching positions. You should therefore actively refine your inner perception and body control over the full range of motion.

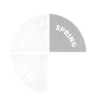

FOR THE SHOULDER AND CHEST: BREAST SHAPING

You will need a dumbbell or weight cuff for this exercise.

❶   This exercise is a good one for women with softer tissue who want to keep their breasts firm. Kneel on all fours, making sure that the hips are over the knees and that the shoulders are over the wrists. Place your palms flat on the mat and press your fingertips slightly into the ground; your arms will automatically rotate to the correct position, and the insides of your elbows should face each other.

❷   Next, gently rotate the upper arm bone outward slightly. Stabilize the position of your lower abdomen and lift one hand off the mat. Take a dumbbell or weight cuff in this hand and swing it under the supporting arm sideways, through to the other side.

Now rock gently in this position; this helps to tighten the connective tissue sheaths of the chest muscles.

After 5–10 repetitions of these seesawing actions, change sides.

The exercises for women on pp. 163-165 are also for gymnastic types.

❶   ❷

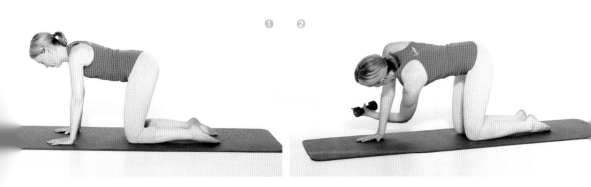

VIKINGS WITH FIRM CONNECTIVE TISSUE

▥ Stretch

You should stretch your fascia often and regularly, using controlled slow expansions and dynamics as well as rocking and finally springs. Stretch often using your body weight or with small dumbbells, and work deliberately to the limit of your elasticity.

▥ Spring

For the spring sector, mainly exercises involving whole-body vibration have been selected, to improve coordination and agility. We concentrate on resilient exercises for stretching the active structures.

▥ Revive

Any activity applied to the fascia that stimulates the metabolism is especially important for you, because your connective tissue tends to become knotted.

▥ Feel

These exercises are suitable for everyone, but more important for less athletic people.

More meaningful exercises for Viking types are the Cat (p. 130), the Eagle Flight (p. 118), and Swinging the Legs (p. 148), as well as the Light Switch Kung Fu Stretch (p. 184). These all increase flexibility and improve coordination, which is particularly important for Viking types.

OPENING UP THE RIBCAGE

Less athletic men in particular tend to lean forward with contracted shoulders. This exercise opens the chest and loosens the stiff structures in this area. Lie down, with your back on a low stool, keeping as flat as you can.

❶ Take a small dumbbell or filled water bottle in each hand. Extend your arms out to the sides. Make sure that your elbow joints are always slightly bent.

❷ Stay in this position and lower your arms using the weight of the dumbbells until the chest feels tight.

❸ Now start to stretch to the extreme in small flexible movements. Use some force, but only as much as feels comfortable. Vary the position of your arms on the sides and over the head by using different angles, and try different hand positions.

❹ Repeat this exercise several times, maintaining slightly bent arms.

❺ – ❻ The Flying Sword (p. 134) is also a very good exercise for both men and women. Please note the advice for people with instability in their back.

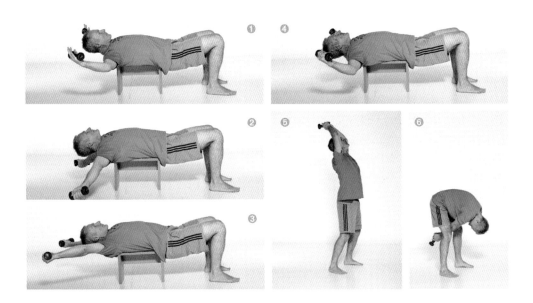

Of Interest to Men and Women

EXERCISES AND TIPS FOR WOMEN

Research and experience have demonstrated that men and women have different problem areas and want to train and shape them in specific ways. There is some evidence that the same principles apply to both sexes with regard to training the fascia.

In fact, in many aspects there are no gender differences: the connective tissue has the same functions in men as in women, although by nature women have slightly softer connective tissue. The exercises in our basic program are therefore well suited to all connective tissue types and to both sexes.

If in the connective tissue test you found out that you are more of a flexible person, you will find the relevant instructions in the corresponding section above. The following exercises aim to address some typical problem areas and needs for both women and men.

There are many women who have soft thighs with unwanted dimpling, but who also suffer from tension in the neck; therefore, the thigh should be tonified and strengthened, and the neck needs to be loosened up. The unwelcome dimples and folds, which commonly exist on the thigh, do not benefit from purely muscle training alone.

The problem lies in the lack of elastic resilience of the superficial fascia, which extends along the outer thigh to below the knee. In this layer, it is common for visible fat deposits and water retention to form the dreaded cellulite. However, regular fascia training with Elastic Jumps and similar exercises improves the collagen density and tissue tonicity in this fascial layer; and this can help to re-introduce a youthful tension on these areas.

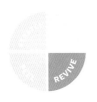

ROLLING OUT THE THIGHS

❶ Proceed as in Rolling Out the Thigh (p. 145).

❷ – ❹ Work over your entire thigh with the roll—the outside, front, back, and inside, as well as the transition to the glutes. Be sure to perform the rotational movement in slow motion.

Think of a sponge from which you want to expel water, so that it can soak up fresh water again.

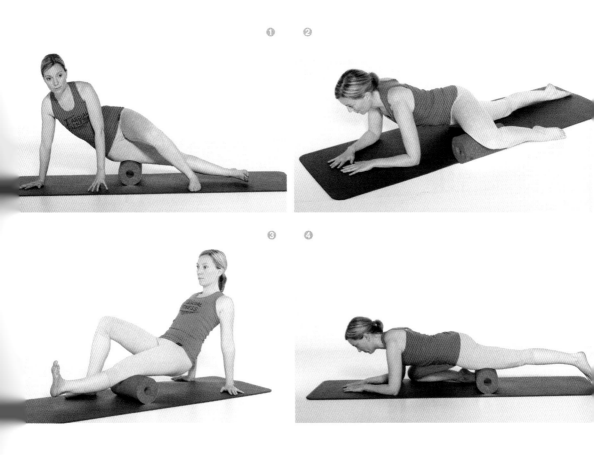

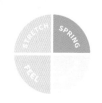

TIGHTENING THE THIGH AND BOTTOM—WITH AND WITHOUT WEIGHTS

This exercise is similar to the Activating the Outer Thigh exercise on p. 146; however, this time we will work on both the inside and the outside of the thigh, and you will be lying on a chair from the start, which stimulates the fascia more comprehensively. If you have problems with your wrists, shoulders, or neck, making the position on the chair difficult for you, then you can perform the exercise on your side on the floor.

It is beneficial to use ankle weights for this exercise. For a woman, an ideal weight to begin with is about 0.75 kg per cuff, but you can progress to heavier weights later if you are comfortable.

❶ Lie sideways on a chair, and hold on to the back of the chair. Start slowly with the upper leg: lift and bend back from the knee. Then change sides and continue with your other leg. This will help to tighten the thigh on both the outside and the inside.

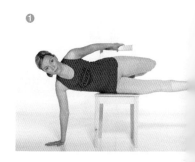

❷ Once you have telescopically stretched your leg, hold this position and pulsate with small, resilient mini-movements upward; this tightens the skin and ensures a nice, firm muscular structure.

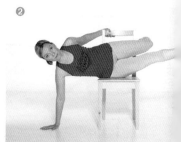

Finally, repeat the exercise again, but without the weight cuff, and enjoy the light and airy feeling in your legs.

FIRMING/TIGHTENING THE TUMMY

❶ Sit upright on the floor or mat, with slightly parted legs and your feet flat. Stretch your arms forward while making sure that your shoulders stay pulled down, as if someone is pulling you forward by your fingers and simultaneously pushing a weight down on your shoulder blades.

❷ – ❸ Next, tilt your pelvis backward, pull your abdominal muscles slightly inward, and roll yourself up and to the side. Make sure that your abdomen remains flat and that your back is curved. Now begin to make small angle changes in the position—tilt a little to the right, then to the left. Rotate your upper body, and roll a little deeper and higher, fluently connecting each position. Now stop and hold this position and gently bounce upward.

Take care and have a rest if you feel uncomfortable or if you are no longer able to keep your back relaxed.

Variation: You can also put a balloon or a ball between your knees during this exercise. Press lightly on the balloon/ball throughout the exercise—this helps to tighten the pelvic floor muscles.

❶   ❷   ❸

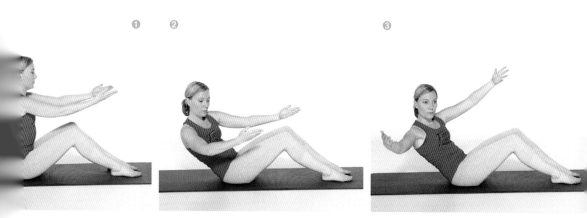

EXERCISES AND TIPS FOR MEN

Men often have shortened structures in their legs, hips, and shoulders, which, if specific to one side, can sometimes be a result of unilateral training. Most of us train for a specific purpose, and everyone wants to look their best in public after all. Men who do weight training should therefore stretch the trained areas in order to balance and maintain their flexibility. This is especially true for those who want to have a strong upper body and wide shoulders.

Some exercises for men for improving elasticity, firmness, and suppleness are given below.

THE FLAMINGO

Stand in front of a chair with your legs hip-width apart. Shift your weight to one side and place your free leg on the seat. Your standing leg should be stable, with the knee kept straight.

❶ Bend your upper body and stretch your arms out over the leg resting on the seat, as far forward as is comfortable. You will feel significant strain on the hamstrings, and so slightly bend your knee in this leg. The angle of bend of the leg on the chair should now be maintained throughout the exercise.

❷ Now vary this tension by gently pushing in and then out a few times, causing the leg to lengthen. Notice the feeling in your back here, as the various stretches usually have an effect on shortened muscle chains. Vary the stretch with small extension and flexing movements of the knee joint. Your stretches should be catlike and supple.

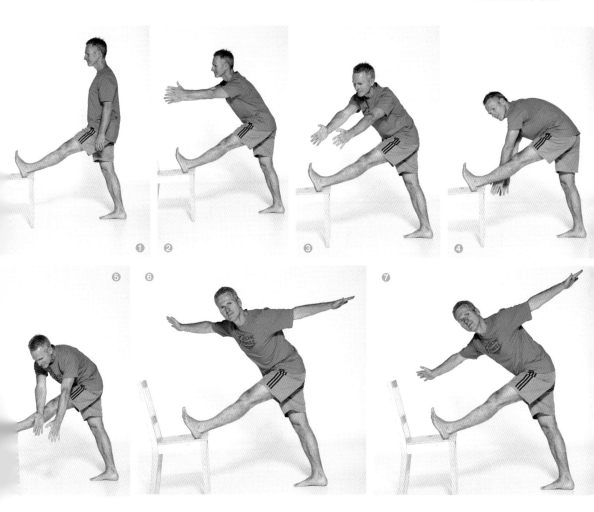

❸ – ❺ You also need to watch your upper body. Pull the tips of your shoulder blades slightly back and down; the sternum should be relaxed and open throughout the leg stretching.

❻ – ❼ Concentrate on this muscle group, starting with the pelvis. Next, try small upper body or pelvis movements and then switch to the fascia chain of the back leg down to the feet. Take your arms forward or to the sides, and pull yourself up in the opposite direction. Try to perform your own stretch and movement actions, from small to large or from basic to more complex. You can playfully and gently stretch out your entire back line (chain).

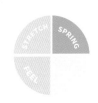

THROWING

❶ In this exercise you simulate a throwing motion, as if you were throwing a ball or a javelin. Try the process of performing a fluid throwing motion without too much force. It is important to preload the torso and arm structures like a rubber band by a countermovement preparatory to the throw. You can hold a ball or convenient object in your hand, without actually throwing it. This activates the brain pattern of movement during practice.

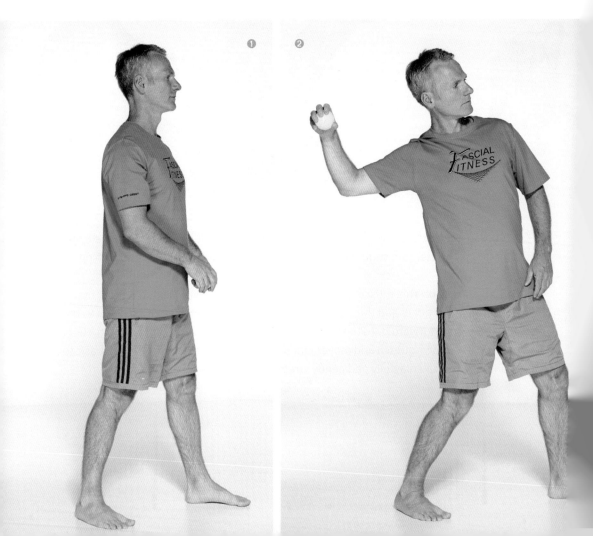

❷ – ❸ Stand straight and pull your arm back in preparation for the throwing action. At this point, the stored energy can be used without great force being necessary for projectile motion. You do not really need to throw—it is all about propulsion. Make sure that the throwing movement impulse comes from the shoulder, and not from the hand like a whipping action. The movement is initiated by the set-up in the shoulder, but then the hand follows through effortlessly like the end of a whip.

Variation (advanced): start the kinetic momentum in front of the sternum and let it flow with a delay from the shoulder and arm, and then to the hand.

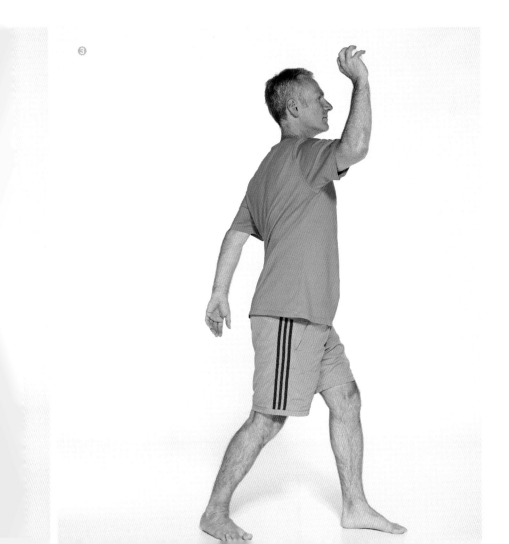

❸

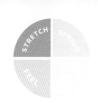
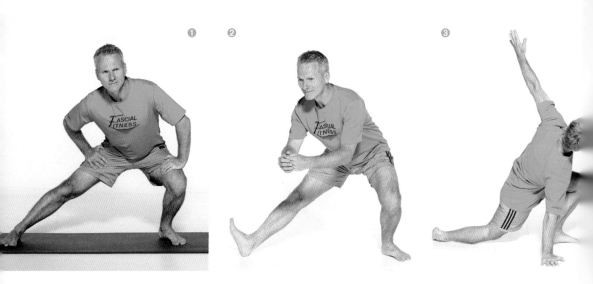

STRETCHING THE ADDUCTORS

❶ This exercise is all about the insides of the thighs, the muscles called the *adductors*, and we will start with a lateral movement. In this position perform gentle rocking movements with the leg which is outstretched, as shown in the image.

❷ Next, transfer the support of the extended leg to the heel and rotate the foot outward. From here make rocking, springing movements with your upper body in different directions.

❸ Now turn the extended leg completely inward, so that the foot rests on the instep. Stretch the opposite arm over the body and back so that the upper body twists slightly. Rock and bounce gently in this position.

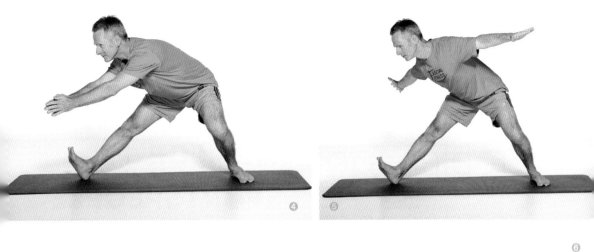

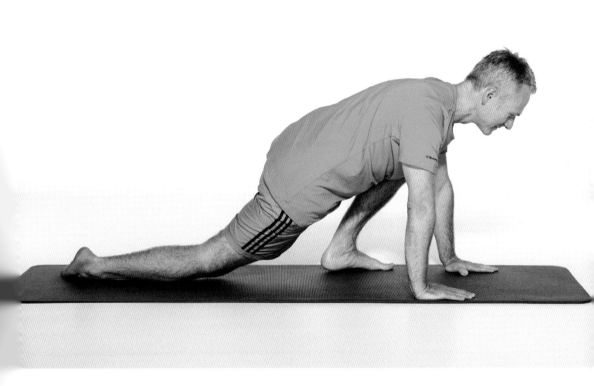

④ – ⑥ Practice all three parts of the exercise on different areas of your body, to optimally stimulate the fascial network.

Another exercise, Opening Up the Ribcage, which is described on p. 161, is also good for many men, especially those undertaking strength training for the upper body.

Problems for Sportspeople

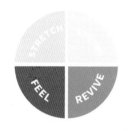

Athletes are by definition well trained, but they still can, and often do, have problems, suffering from restricted movement, stiffness, or pain. These conditions often occur as a result of unbalanced training as well as injuries or excessive strain. New knowledge and research regarding the fascia could contribute to a better understanding in the future, whether this is the involvement of the fascia in sore muscles, or the realization that connective tissue in good condition helps prevent injuries. In the majority of sports injuries it is the white fascia that is affected and not the muscles. What also has a strong impact is new knowledge about the elastic storage capability of the fascia, which is drawn on in various forms of training.

In certain sports some fascial and muscular problems occur repeatedly; these will be covered in this section. Those of you who want to explore this subject can consult the sports science literature. For more information, see the Appendix.

TIPS FOR SPORTSPEOPLE

Flexibility is especially relevant to all athletes (though to some more than others), and the mobility of our collagen structures is more important than that of the contractile ones, namely the red muscle fibers. The fascial tissue—tendons, muscle cases, and joint capsules—has to be maintained, and the appropriate fascia training is a must for athletes. It is essential to do regular exercise that stimulates these tissues and increases the muscle's facility of perception.

Begin each workout in your sport with the fascia exercises from the revive sector, such as rolling out the structures that you particularly require (e.g. the thighs, calves, feet, and back). Start your training by rolling out at a slightly faster pace, so that the muscles will be stimulated and warmed up. The rolling-out exercises after a workout or competition should be completed at a slower speed.

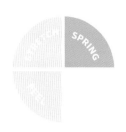

The next section explains how to address sore muscles (p. 173); see also the exercises in the sections for the back (pp. 128-137), and for the hip and thighs (pp. 144-150). A slow rolling-out is relaxing and stimulates tissue regeneration; more discussion of this will follow in the next section.

Anyone who undertakes strength training should always stretch the trained areas of muscle sufficiently to compensate for muscle tightening and to achieve flexibility. For golfers, tennis players, and participants in other ball and racket sports, the storage capacity of the tendons in the shoulders and arms is important. In this case the throwing exercise on p. 168 is very beneficial.

SELF-HELP FOR SORE MUSCLES

A short self-help program for sore muscles comprises rolling out with the fascia roll and slow stretching. The rolling-out is like a self-massage; a real massage would be even better, of course, but more of a luxury. Adjust the pressure when rolling, so that you experience no more than a light squeezing; a pleasant feeling will then arise in the tired connective tissue.

The following exercises are good for sore muscles: slow, gentle stretching, as in the Elephant Step described below (p. 178) and the Cat (p. 130); the Flamingo (p. 166); and the Eagle Flight (p. 118). Below, you will find recommendations for more stretching exercises, depending on the muscles concerned (p. 178).

1. Rolling Out the Calves

2. Rolling Out Other Body Parts

3. Slow Stretching for Sore Muscles: the Elephant Step

ROLLING OUT THE CALVES

Position the roller under the calf, approximately at the level of the Achilles tendon. The other leg needs to rest on the mat to help control the pressure.

❶ Raise your buttocks up, and start slowly and carefully to put weight onto the contact points. Use small, tentative movements for this exercise, letting the roller slowly travel one millimeter at a time up the calf.

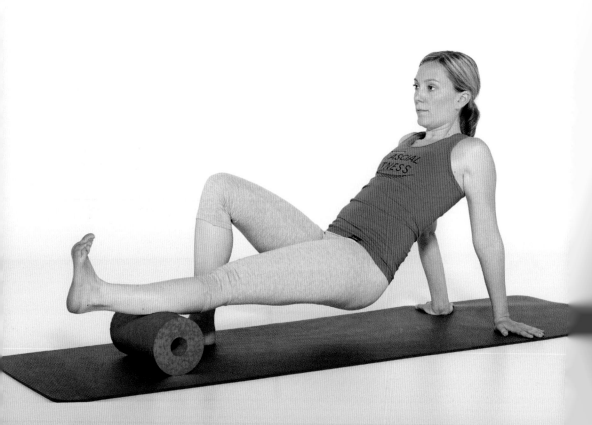

❷ Do this exercise in slow motion. If the pressure is too painful, then keep your pelvis on the mat. If you want to increase the pressure, you can lift up the other leg as an additional weight to the lower leg on the roll.

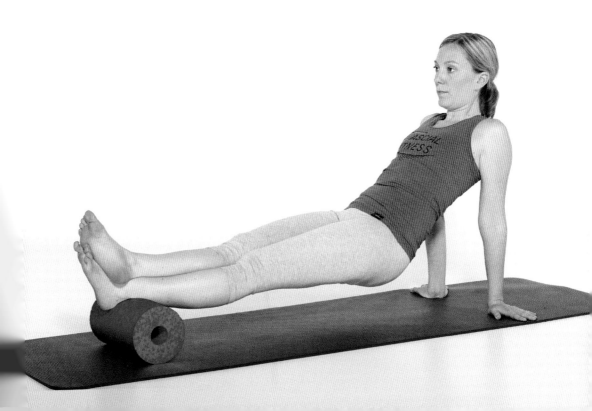

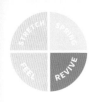

ROLLING OUT OTHER BODY PARTS

This slow, relaxing rolling-out procedure covers many parts of the body, including the thighs (p. 145, 163) and the back (p. 128), and, using balls and smaller rolls, the forearms (p. 141) and the chest and upper body.

❶ Rolling out the pectorals and fascia with a tennis ball.

❷ Rolling out the chest and arms with the fascia roll.

❸ Rolling out the back and lumbar fascia.

❹ Rolling out the outer thigh.

❺ Rolling out the front thigh.

❻ Rolling out the hamstrings—note here the crossed leg. This creates a bit of pressure on the back leg, so make appropriate adjustments so that it is comfortable for you.

❼ – ❽ Rolling out the forearms with a small fascia roll or with a filled water bottle.

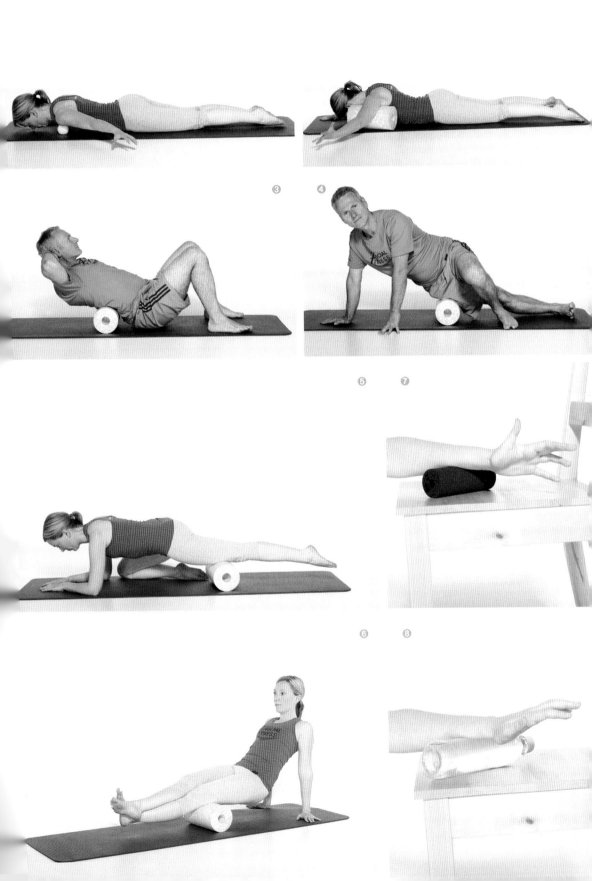

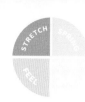
SLOW STRETCHING FOR SORE MUSCLES: THE ELEPHANT STEP

❶ Start from the all-fours position. Make sure that the hips are over the knees and that the shoulders are over the wrists. Keep your hands flat on the mat and press the fingertips slightly into the ground; your arms will then automatically rotate into the correct position, and the insides of your elbows will face each other.

Next, rotate the humerus gently outward. Tighten the lower abdomen and slightly lift your bottom into the air until you end up in a comfortable spanning triangle position. Then bring the pelvis all the way back down, and lower your heels as far as possible toward the mat.

❷ Now bend your knees one after the other, as in the Cat (p. 130), alternating one leg at a time.

❸ – ❹ Next, move your feet slowly, step by step, toward your hands. As you do this, your buttocks will rise even higher—the angle formed by your body will become more acute.

Once you have reached your maximum, walk your hands forward, step by step, until you return to the starting position.

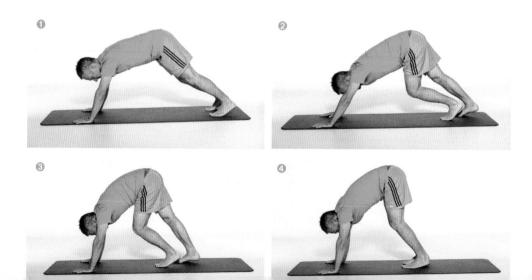

BALANCING EXERCISES FOR RUNNERS

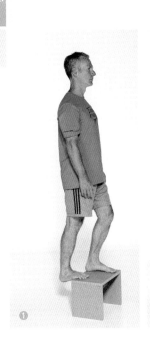 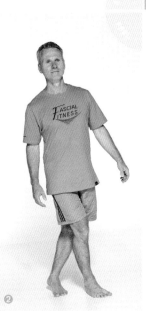 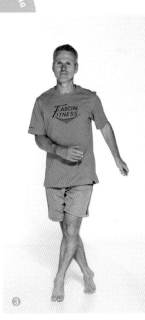 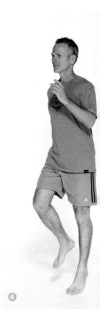

① It is important for runners to stretch the heavily stressed Achilles tendon in order to keep it supple and to increase elasticity and storage capacity. The stretching exercise for the Achilles tendon is described on p. 156.

② – ④ It is beneficial to vary the training for your running. This is especially true in the case of endurance runners; they move more uniformly and should therefore vary the movement patterns in their training. Try the following: change direction, walk backward or sideways, do cross overs, or add a couple of hops.

As you run, obstructions such as banks or obstacles on the walkway force you to automatically vary your movement, for example jumping light footed in your running rhythm, up and down again. Stay lively and agile, so that you train your body awareness and the fascia while running optimally. You will also subject the joints and tendons to a new load angle.

INSTRUCTIONS FOR CYCLISTS

Cyclists only use certain parts of their body while riding—the calves, thighs, and hips—and the movement sequence is always the same. The knee and hip joints are strained, within a very small radius, on one side only—the back. The backs of the thighs are often shortened in cyclists, and the structures above the knees and the hips are sometimes less mobile.

Uneven loading: the long fascia track of the back line is sometimes reduced or overstretched in cyclists.

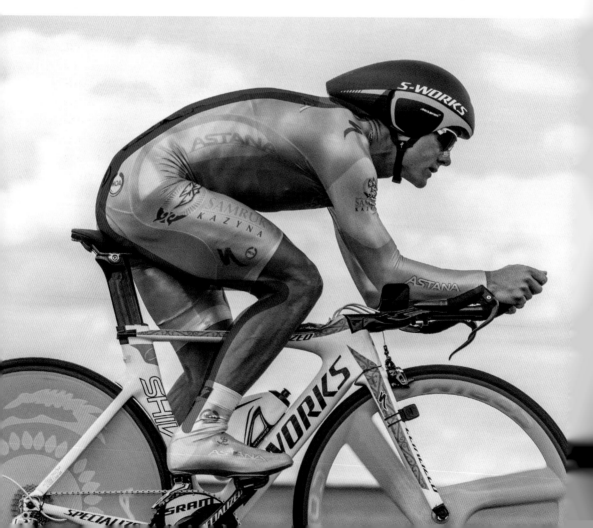

STRETCH

In my experience, participants in the Tour de France and other long cycling races suffer for quite a few days after their event: they become extremely stiff, which is probably because of the one-sided impact. Therefore, if you only train specific muscles for your activity, it is not just that particular muscle group that is affected, but also the entire muscle fascia unit. Commonly, a swelling can occur in the muscle tissue, but, more specifically, there can be liquid congestion; however, in the long run the red muscle can actually be shortened through one-sided training.

Cyclists should therefore consciously compensate by regularly performing stretching exercises, such as the Cat (p. 130) and the Eagle Flight (p. 118). Stretches for the chest in the Viking exercise section (p. 160) are also recommended, because the upper body of a cyclist typically adopts a contracted position. This leads to the superficial back line being unevenly balanced and loaded; the combination of this on extended road trips and intensive training has an adverse effect in the long term. The backs of the thighs become burdened and shortened down to below the knees. The back of the neck, and the entire rear portions of muscle groups, are constantly being stretched at the same time.

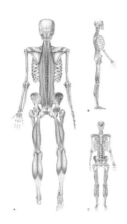

The superficial back line.

Everyday Life as an Exercise

MORE-CREATIVE MOVEMENTS!

Our goal here is more-creative activity in everyday life. Use your full range of motion in your standard movements, in order to become more versatile and relaxed. Day-to-day body movements put demands on and stimulate your fascia, and also ensure the full use of your joints. This is important, as these movements keep the musculoskeletal system healthy, which does not have to depend on exercise via a specific training program or sport.

Here we will try some exercises that you can do on a casual basis whenever you have the inclination—you do not need to change into sports clothes. Just take a few minutes to do these stretches whenever you feel the need. This will help to break up your routine, and you will feel refreshed after the activity. Try a few of the Stair Dance steps at the office, or perform the Light Switch Kung Fu Stretch and African Bending at any time of day.

1. The Stair Dance

2. Light Switch Kung Fu Stretch

3. African Bending in Everyday Life

THE STAIR DANCE

❶ – ❺ Staircases offer the chance to do a short fascia training exercise. Jump lightly in control and as softly as possible from step to step, and vary the positions of your feet. Turn inward and outward, and jump to the right and left of the stairs, as well as up and down, keeping the movements controlled and quiet.

In the Stair Dance, you can practice barefoot or with flexible shoes; however, heeled shoes would not be suitable. The movements should be dance-like and playful, and performed in a casual fashion. Ideally, the Stair Dance should become a habit on the stairs.

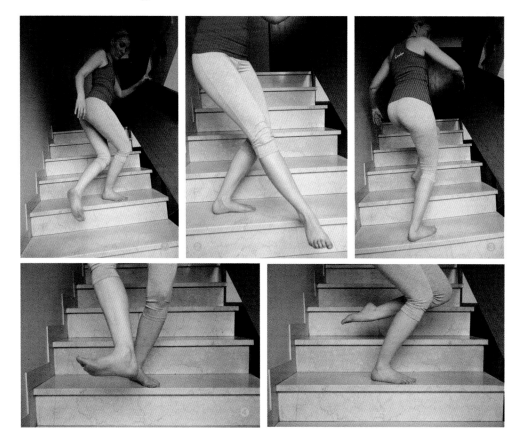

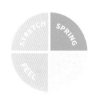

LIGHT SWITCH KUNG FU STRETCH

You will need confidence for this exercise, but you can really have fun doing it. While we don't suggest you act like the Karate Kid in real life, this exercise has some similarities to a Martial Arts kick and needs to be controlled. So, instead of switching the light on with your hand, use your toes. Practice with care to avoid damaging the wallpaper!

❶ Prepare to switch the light on with your toes: assume a side-step stance and get ready to kick with your back foot.

❷ – ❸ Aim your chosen foot at the switch and try to hit it. More advanced users can also rotate and hit the switch by standing with their back to the wall. You may also look out for some door handles which you could start to touch with a gentle foot-kick in the future rather than your habitual hand-touching style.

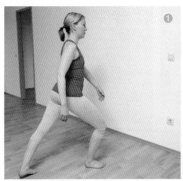
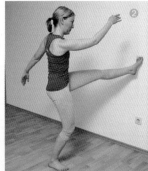
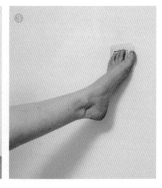

AFRICAN BENDING IN EVERYDAY LIFE

Whenever you pick something up off the floor you initiate the upward movement by bouncing dynamically downwards first. A comfortable way to accomplish this, and a good exercise, is the African technique (see p. 132). Arch deeply from the lumbar region, take a brief pause here, then bounce once or twice using the full range of motion.

Guidelines for the Elderly

Aging changes the fascia, especially since many older people become less active over time, and if you do not move very much, your fascia becomes dry and brittle. For older people, fascia training is therefore particularly important. Here are some tips specifically for people over 60.

Regeneration of the connective tissue still works, but the process slows down as you get older. Regular rolling and stimulating the fascia with exercises from the revive sector encourage fascia metabolism and help to maintain the tissue.

In everyday life, flexibility and coordination are particularly important for general mobility and for avoiding falls; therefore, choose exercises from the sector that includes stretching and feeling.

Strengthening exercises referred to in the spring sector are suitable for the fitter group of people who want to maintain their level of fitness. Although you do not need to generate an excessive amount of power, you should still exercise with greater care.

A good exercise, for example, is the Swinging Bamboo (p. 142), or try the Flying Sword (p. 134) for a good full-body exercise; be sure to perform these gently. Start slowly and avoid any jerky, dynamic actions—let your breathing dictate the flow of movement.

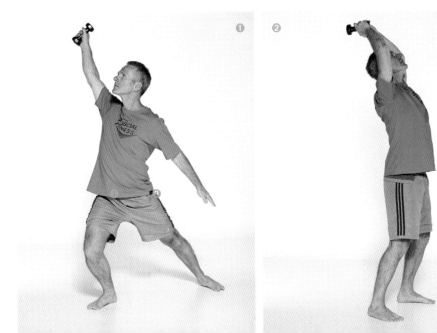

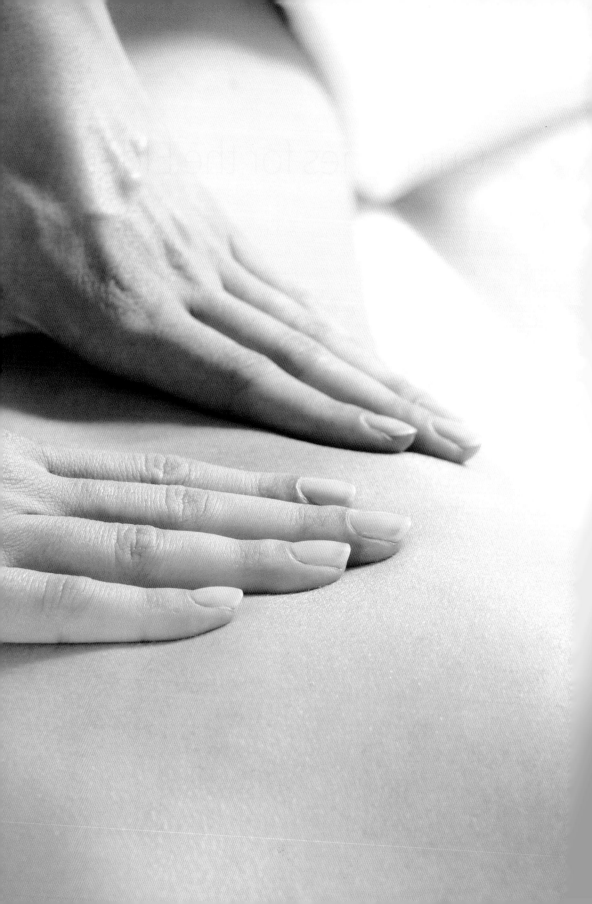

CHAPTER 4

Fascia, Physiotherapy, & Gentle Healing Methods

Fascia, physiotherapy, and natural movement remedies are closely connected. Physiotherapy is possibly the field in which new findings from fascia research are emerging the most frequently, but perhaps even entire theoretical models will need to be re-evaluated. Physiotherapists at various levels are also fascia specialists—in 2007, at the first international Fascia Congress at Harvard University, invitations were therefore extended to physiotherapists in addition to physicians and biologists. Throughout their years of experience of direct manual contact with the body, and its reaction, many physiotherapists have accumulated useful knowledge that can be of benefit in fascia research. My own training as a Rolfer and Feldenkrais teacher fills me with enduring inspiration and questions for the scientific exploration of fascial tissue dynamics.

In this chapter I would like to explain some consequences of the new knowledge gained from fascia research, relating to some manual and other so-called *alternative therapies*. I find this area very interesting and it has opened up several avenues to integrative and complementary therapy strategies. The procedures on which I comment here concern the teaching of movement, as well as manual therapies. Knowledge about the healing properties of gymnastics and massage has been chronicled throughout the years. It is likely that the origins of gymnastics and massage as curative methods date back to the Stone Age. Forms of these can be found in many cultures: China, which has one of the world's oldest exercise cultures, has been reporting activities regarding physical exercises and manual loading since the 4th millennium BC, and the established practices in India, which has the oldest systematic medicine tradition in the world, are well known. Massage is today part of folk medicine. In European medicine and culture, especially those of ancient Greece and Rome, there have been strong traditions of physical exercise and massage, both in sport and in the art of healing. The fact that massage has a calming effect and promotes healing has been medically confirmed.

This knowledge became somewhat neglected in the European Middle Ages, but made a comeback during the Renaissance, and then after the Age of Enlightenment it truly blossomed. In the 19th century especially, there was almost a continental movement in physical education— the Swedish "father of gymnastics" Per Henrik Ling as well as his German counterpart Friedrich Ludwig Jahn come to mind here. Manual procedures were extensively promoted during this period through natural medicine, with particular acceptance of this influence in Germany. A second wave occurred from the 1920s to the 1950s. In 1970 a brand-new boom

in gentle Eastern and alternative methods reached us: yoga, shiatsu, acupuncture, qigong, Pilates, and much more.

Nowadays, some of the success of these various methods can be more clearly explained on the basis of the fascia research that has been carried out, and they can now be seen in a new light. So-called *soft* or *complementary* procedures actually often had effects that we were unable to explain in the past; this applies to a variety of procedures, including acupuncture, yoga, osteopathy, and Pilates. The original underlying theories

Over the centuries, doctors have acknowledged the effects of massage.

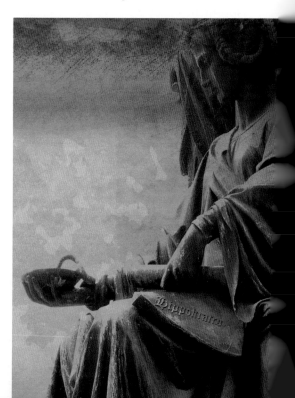

of life energy, meridians, blockages, or disturbed harmony derived from traditional knowledge, sometimes intuitive insights, or simply speculation. Esoteric concepts, however, could not convince previously skeptical doctors and scientists, myself included. You know my side of the story already, but some clinical success has been acknowledged for these methods without any plausible explanations for the positive results.

As we now know, a more plausible explanation for many of the observed beneficial properties of these therapeutic modalities can be found in the various functions of the fascia: stretch deformation and sensory stimulation, liquid exchange, metabolism, and its interaction with the nervous system. Many manual methods and forms of exercise more or less systematically reach the fascia. It might be a surprise to some of the traditional teachers in these modalities that these methods actually influence the fascia, which could explain some of their known achievements and scientific effects. I will explain by using some selected examples.

YOGA

This ancient Indian exercise technique has been developing over many centuries. As far back as 700 BC at least, it was described in the older Upanishads, a collection of texts containing philosophical concepts of Hinduism. Originally, yoga consisted of a series of aesthetic exercises, which helped meditation by influencing the breathing rhythm. In the original sense of Hindu yoga, it had a spiritual framework, and is embedded in a tradition of self-discipline and renunciation. It is not a sports program but belongs to the search for enlightenment and the desire for self-development. The known forms of yoga in the West, however, include some fairly stressful exercises and are quite different from their Indian origins, although many exercises and positions are still based on the original forms.

The acknowledged success of yoga exercises in the treatment of pain, and specifically back pain, has been the subject of study by experts over the last 20 years. Yoga has been proven to reduce stress and regulate excessively high blood pressure. International scientific studies, including one from Germany by Professor Andreas Michalsen (a natural medicine researcher in Berlin), have confirmed these results. The reason for such positive achievements is mainly believed to be that yoga has a psychological effect, as it uses specific body poses for long periods and reduces stress by remaining in one position. Meditation and the spiritual aspect of yoga will particularly help because they activate self-healing powers.

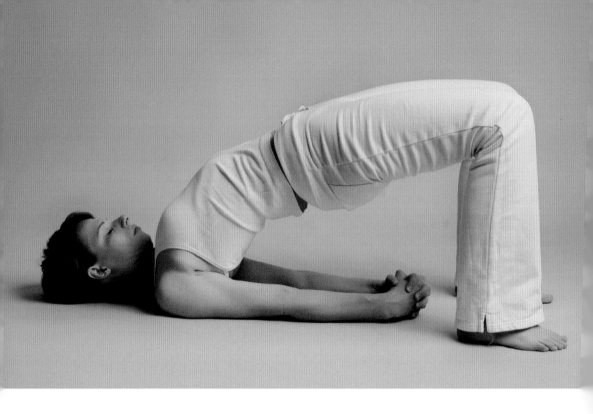

Poses from ancient India are now being reinterpreted.

Muscle strengthening and improved circulation have also been attributed to yoga. The standard explanation for these effects of the physical exercises is as follows. Yoga consists mainly of stretching exercises in positions that are held for long periods. These stretches clearly reach the fascia: among other effects, the stretches cause the fascia to react with signals to the central nervous system which is able to alter the resting muscle tone in the body as well as balancing the basic tuning of the autonomous nervous system. It is likely that these reactions in the fascia are responsible for most of the positive physical effects.

Helene Langevin is one of the most respected neuroscientists; she has held the chair of complementary and integrative medicine at the Osher Institute of Harvard Medical School, among other positions. She has investigated, using scientific methods, the effectiveness and applicability of alternative health treatments. In animal experiments, Langevin proved that static stretching is able to reduce inflammation. To do this, a substance was injected into the deep fascia of the back of rats, which caused inflammation: as a result, the animals' movements were tense and they showed symptoms of back pain. Some of the treated rats were then stretched gently by hand for 10 minutes daily over 12 days. This was designed to simulate the strains encountered during yoga practice. The result was that the rats which underwent the manual stretching recovered their normal movement much faster and their inflammation subsided more rapidly. Tissue samples taken later showed that there were fewer inflammatory cells in the treated rats' back fascia than in that of the untreated rats.

An extensive clinical study of human back pain patients carried out by a student of Helene Langevin subsequently revealed that stretching may actually explain the benefits of yoga for these patients.

A large number of patients were asked to participate in another research program by Karen Sherman at the University of Seattle. These patients were divided into three groups: the first took up yoga as part of a conventional back exercise program, including stretching, for three months; the second read a self-help book about pain; and the third carried out exercises for breathing and meditation, as well as receiving tips on lifestyle. The result was that the group with the self-help book showed very little benefit, whereas both the yoga and the gym exercise groups demonstrated almost the same level of success in terms of reporting less pain. This study has been documented internationally, and it is regarded now as evidence that yoga alone, or in combination with meditation and spiritual activity, tends to have beneficial effects on low back pain.

Nevertheless, the detailed mechanics of how exactly these positive stretching effects are accomplished – to what degree the tissue is loosened, which cytokines or neurotransmitters are secreted, and what exact changes in the nervous system are triggered – still remains to be clarified. More research should, and will, continue in this area, of course, but these more up-to-date explanatory models about the fascial effect from yoga and about the role of fascia in back pain are very promising.

MASSAGE AND MANUAL THERAPY

Massage is probably the oldest healing method in the world. Throughout history, specially trained slaves have given massages to competitors such as Olympic athletes and gladiators; their success was gauged primarily by the achievement of better blood circulation and of the general relaxation of muscles.

The fascia probably played an important role, because massage stimulates the fascia metabolism and distributes neurotransmitters and hormones, and it is part of a specific system for social bonding and stress regulation that our species shares with other primates.

Massage using a slow, rhythmic pressure also promotes the exchange of fluids in the fascia, as we have already discussed. Inflammatory substances and metabolic waste products

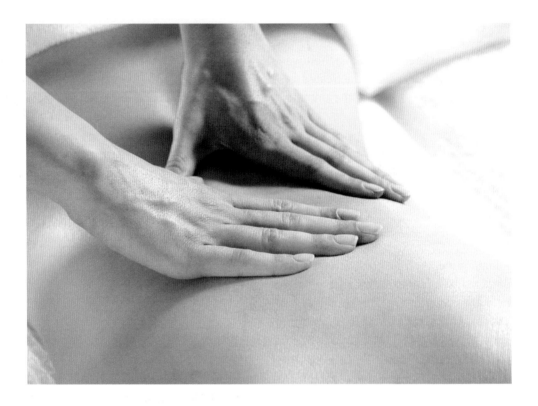

Healing with the hands goes back a long way.

– which are increasingly accumulated during stressful periods – are therefore removed from the connective tissues during massage, which will subsequently refill with fresh fluid and nutrients. In addition, massage leads to the secretion of anti-inflammatory messenger substances in the skin and the fascia; these substances can resolve stickiness and resistance issues in the fascia, as fascia researchers have demonstrated. Remember the massaging of post-surgical scars on the abdomen in the animal trial by Geoffrey Bove and Susan Chapelle, mentioned in Chapter 2 (see p. 42). Incidentally, these animals were massaged using slow, gentle, flowing movements similar to the techniques that are applied in Rolfing. Some of the biochemical and neuro-reflex effects of massage have long been known in physiology. Notwithstanding, the fact that fascial properties are probably involved to at least a similar degree as the muscles and their blood supply, provides a new dimension.

ACUPUNCTURE

Acupuncture is a complementary therapy and undoubtedly helps with back and knee pain. But why? The Chinese have used needles in the bodies of patients since about the 2nd century BC. Life energy is alleged to flow along pathways, described as meridians, throughout the whole body. If these meridians become blocked, then the insertion of needles will free them again. Yin and yang are an additional philosophical concept, representing female and male energies.

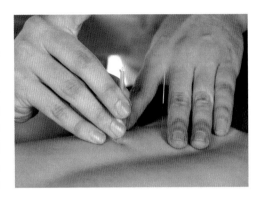

Needles in the skin to combat pain: **acupuncture actually works.**

A total of 400 acupuncture points can be stimulated and brought into balance. However, the existence of negative energies and energetically charged meridians, through which all life energy flows, are not a scientifically-proven concept to satisfy modern Western medical scientists. Nevertheless, acupuncture obviously works, and in her investigations of complementary procedures Helene Langevin has demonstrated a part played by the fascia. The acupuncture points are actually located on specific meeting lines between fascial membranes, which are themselves equipped with receptors and are able react with reflex responses. The receptors send signals to the brain as well as the muscles if they are stimulated (by needles, but also by pressure and massage). In other words, acupuncture needles stimulate a reaction from the fascia, so that a healing effect is produced.

ROLFING

You should already be aware of this method of manual treatment, because we mentioned it in the discussion of the pioneers of fascia research in Chapter 1. Scientific studies of Rolfing mainly originate in the United States, but the potential benefits of this technique have so far not been widely recognized by official Health Authorities. My colleagues in this field are currently busy documenting the clinical effectiveness of this modality for back and shoulder pain, general soft tissue pain, as well as for several posture problems.

The original idea was that a Rolfing therapist could plastically deform the connective tissue by the pure mechanical pressure from the treating hands in order to realign it in its original shape and tonicity. Ida P. Rolf was, in many respects, correct in a large number of her original concepts. She was a genuine pioneer in this new area, with the intention of understanding and fostering the proper functioning of the fascial network for human performance.

Some of Ida Rolf's explanations, however, appear obsolete from today's perspective, such as the idea that you can permanently deform dense fibrous connective tissues using manual pressure for a few seconds or minutes only. Moreover, she did not know that fascia is the home of millions of sensory nerve endings, but instead regarded it as an interesting mechanical material. Had she been able to experience the rapid pace of modern fascia research, I am convinced she would be just as enthusiastic as her therapist colleagues of today. Anyway, her findings and her manual techniques have

Rolfing manual techniques reach deep into the tissue and directly target the fascia.

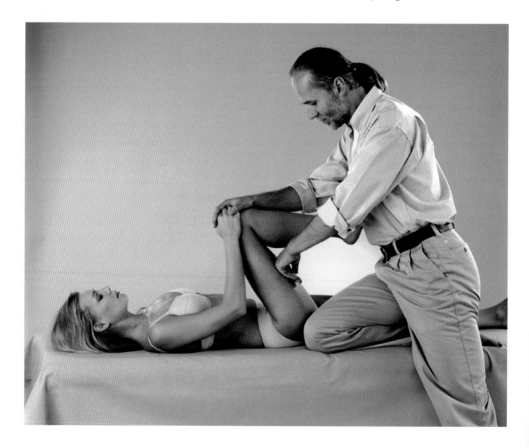

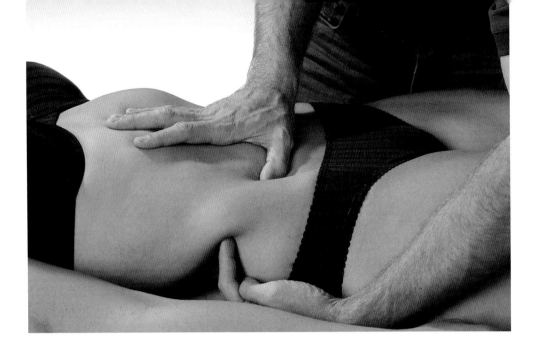

Osteopaths now strongly support their methods by using their knowledge of the fascia.

proved effective; this, among other things, was demonstrated in a study of a series of ten Rolfing sessions for patients with neck pain.

Rolfing techniques consist of slow, gentle massage strokes and very firm manipulation of the fascia of the bodies of muscle in regions such as the lumbar spine, shoulders, and neck. There are also effects on the shoulders and arms through exercise and stretching using these techniques, as well as special techniques for lifting the pelvis and thus involving the long fascial chains.

OSTEOPATHY

Osteopathy is a manual process which includes treatments for virtually all diseases. You read a little about this topic in Chapter 1 (see p. 43) and about its founder Andrew Taylor Still. After his death, osteopathy was further developed in different directions during the 20th century.

Today's osteopaths strongly reinforce their methods with knowledge of the fascia. The treatment is performed by the hands of the therapist using certain grips and massage techniques. Osteopathic treatments, however, are somewhat controversial. According to studies carried out by the Osteopath Association, the treatments do work for many pain symptoms and specific regulatory problems, such as high blood pressure, migraine, and chronic diseases.

Osteopathy is accepted by some health insurance companies, although as yet neither the theoretical background nor its physiological mechanism has been clearly proven, despite a fair amount of documented research. Nevertheless, osteopathy is very popular; it continues to receive growing recognition by health authorities and to be investigated with larger clinical trials.

The method is based on the concept that all the organs and parts of the body are in motion, because they are components of a living, working, liquid system. And indeed there is a body-wide exchange of fluids over the fascia network; moreover, the movement of large muscles and organs is crucially dependent on smooth functioning within their fascial envelopes.

The achievements in osteopathy could be due to the manual stimulation of the fascia, whereby its metabolism is in turn stimulated or neural reflexes and reactions are induced. Some of the effectiveness of osteopathic treatments can be supported with scientific proof, which explains the role of the fascia—however, this proof is not yet comprehensive.

Osteopaths offer a solution for so many problems, although the techniques are not consistent. But it seems clear that the beneficial effect rely to a considerable extent on the participation of the fascia. Some scientists, including the Italian physiotherapy researcher and osteopath Paolo Tozzi (who was a participant at our Fascia Congresses), are strongly focusing their current investigations on the fascial effects of specific osteopathic techniques.

PILATES

The body and movement program known as *Pilates* was developed by a professional boxer and circus artist—Joseph Hubert Pilates—who, not by chance, had a solid sports background. He was born in 1883 in Mönchengladbach, Germany, and emigrated to England in 1912; later, in the United States, his method of training evolved into a Pilates program for soldiers and police officers. As a prisoner of war during the First World War, he kept his fellow prisoners fit through exercise. Apparently, thanks to Pilates, the POWs had a better rate of survival than many others during the great flu epidemic of 1918 to 1920. Joseph Pilates subsequently developed his program in a medical gymnastics and rehabilitation direction, as training for dancers. He worked in the United States with Rudolf von Laban, who we mentioned briefly in Chapter 2 (see p. 69).

Today, Pilates is very popular, because it includes dance and playful elements and comprises both stretching and strengthening; in particular, it improves coordination. This is not surprising, as the movements have some basis in circus acrobatics. The focus is on strengthening the body core—the abdominal, hip, and pelvic muscles—which is referred to as the *powerhouse* in Pilates language. The benefits of this strengthening for treating back pain are well proven, but the Pilates method has also demonstrated success in addressing many other pain syndromes as well as stress and regulation issues.

Joseph Pilates explained the effectiveness of the training method in terms of "springs" and "slings" in the body; as a non-medical professional, he almost certainly meant the fascia in this description, without specifically naming it. He probably had an astute sense of body movement and anatomy, and hence an intuitive understanding of the participation of the muscular connective tissue and the large fascial chains.

Typical Pilates exercises strengthen the body's core.

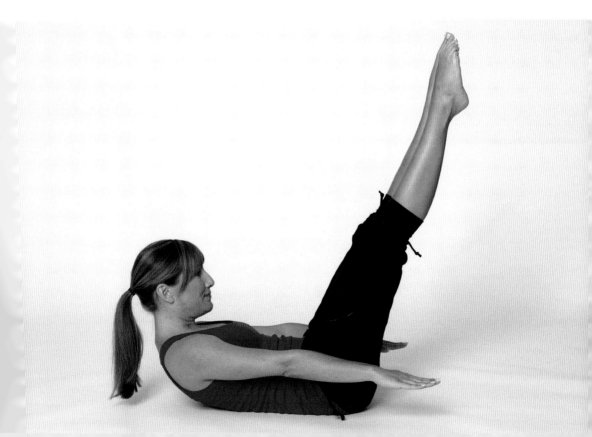

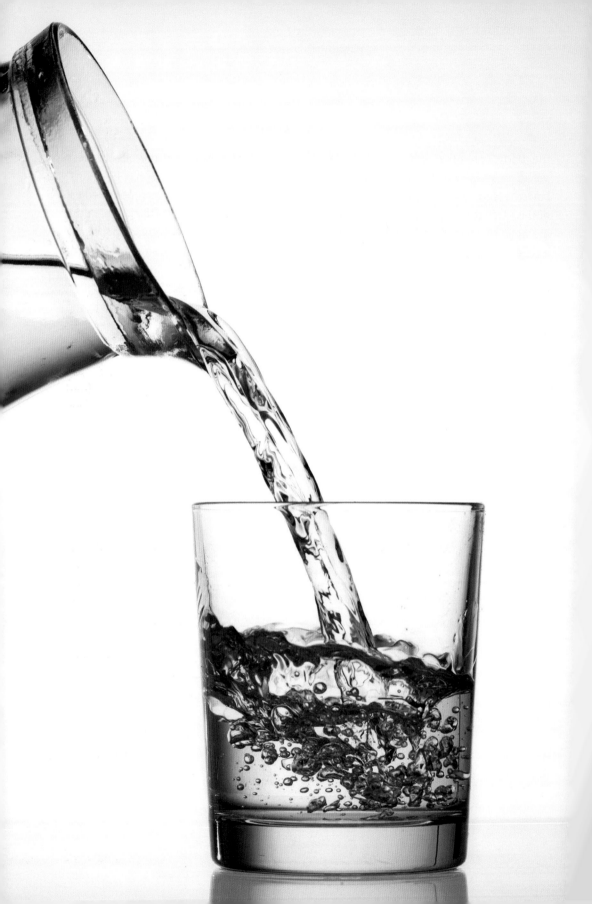

CHAPTER 5

Fit Fascia: Diet and Healthy Lifestyle

This short chapter is dedicated to the subject of diet and lifestyle. Frequently asked questions about food are: What should we eat? How does nutrition affect the fascia? Which minerals, trace elements, or vitamins are important?

In general, a healthy diet and lifestyle clearly help to keep your fascia fit or restore its fitness. This is almost self-evident, as ultimately the maintenance of the whole body depends on nutritious food and sufficient sleep. The most helpful advice is already well known and does not need to be added to; however, there are a few aspects which deserve special attention and which you can optimize if you really want to maintain a healthy fascia.

The tips given here are based on well-known food and health advice, and not on comprehensive nutritional recommendations—only the information that is specifically important for the fascia is emphasized. A few personal tips are included at the end.

MAINTAIN A HEALTHY WEIGHT

Try to avoid being clearly overweight, as carrying too much weight means that the subsystems of the bones, joints, ligaments, tendons, and fascia will be under more pressure. In addition, you may suffer from greatly reduced mobility. Excess weight has an effect on the adipose tissue in particular, which is a part of the fascia, where much more fat will be stored; moreover, the fat cells release unfavorable hormones, as well as many inflammatory substances, all of which have proven harmful effects on our metabolism and fascia. Cosmetically, being overweight also often increases the visibility of cellulite on the tummy, legs, bottom, and upper arms.

DON'T SMOKE

It is a known fact that smoking damages the whole body, and if you really want to improve the health of your fascia, then you should not smoke at all. Smoking results in considerable cellular damage, and free radicals in the body cause the oxygen content of the blood to decline dramatically. In addition, the inhalation of nicotine poisons the blood vessels, constricting them and causing stress. The end result is that the fascia receives fewer nutrients. It has been proved that smokers have a greater risk of back pain, cartilage damage, osteoarthritis, and herniated discs, all of which are connected with a poor supply of fibrous structures.

Excess weight puts more pressure not only on the bones, but also on the fascia.

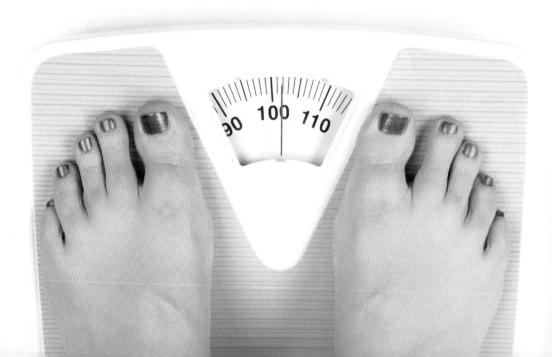

KEEP HYDRATED

The fascia consists of almost 70% water, and it needs a plentiful supply—the general advice is to drink one to one and a half liters of water a day. Our system needs fresh plain water, which means that juices, lemonade, colas, milk-based drinks, and coffee are not included. These are all stimulants, and not reliable for quenching the tissue thirst for clean water. It is better to accustom yourself to drinking tap water without carbonation—it is, after all, widely available. In competitive sports you may choose to drink more water or alternative drinks; however, do not drink these in large quantities, as excessive liquid consumption can be harmful too.

PROTEIN IS IMPORTANT

Protein fibers form the most important basic material of the fascia; to manufacture these fibers our body itself has need of protein. Essential amino acids must come from food, as our body cannot create them naturally. For the production of connective tissue cell fibers, an adequate intake of protein is therefore necessary. Animal protein tends to provide more comprehensive nutrition than vegetable protein—eating high-quality meat, eggs, dairy products, and fish, is therefore an easy way to give the body what it needs. In the case of vegetarians, it is particularly important to know about lentils, beans, or other legumes, and to be aware of which

Our entire metabolism requires water—it is particularly important for connective tissue.

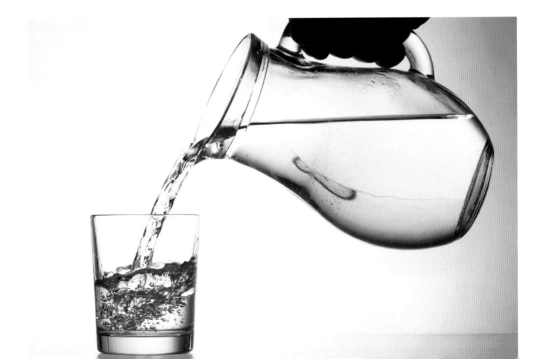

dairy products have enough protein. It is wise to familiarize yourself with good cookery books and consult scientific nutrient tables regarding sources of protein.

VITAMIN C FOR COLLAGEN

The synthesis of collagen in the connective tissue depends on vitamin C—the cells need it as a kind of "glue," to keep the fibers all together. The absence of vitamin C in the body leads to symptoms of tissue deficiency, because collagen production is disrupted. Some examples of these issues are dental gum bleeding, poor wound healing, detachment of bone skin, and calluses, as well as other ailments such as scurvy. Vitamin C is very important for the connective tissue. A genuine lack of this vitamin is quite rare, but do pay attention to it.

Did you know that fruit is not the best source of vitamin C? The amount in apples and lemons and oranges is less than in fresh vegetables; have a look at a vitamin table for confirmation. Varieties of cabbage—such as broccoli, Brussel sprouts, and kale—contain more vitamin C than citrus fruits. Spinach, fennel, parsley, chili peppers, and especially bell peppers are also high in vitamin C; even potatoes are reliable sources of this vitamin. In the summer, strawberries and other native berries are available sources. Tropical

Meat and dairy products provide a great deal of valuable protein, and vegetarians need to be aware of the benefits of lentils, beans, or other legumes.

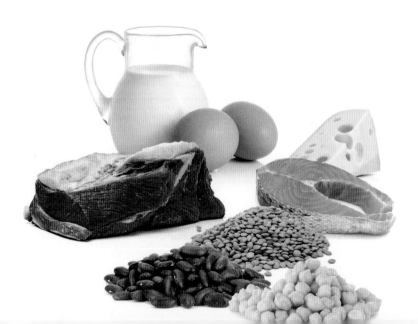

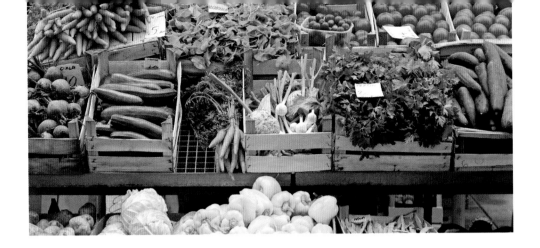

Cabbages and peppers are good sources of vitamin C.

fruits—such as kiwis, guava, papaya, and acerola berries (processed)—in juice or powder form are also very rich in vitamin C. A variety of fresh vegetables, however, is the most economical way of getting this most important vitamin.

ZINC, MAGNESIUM, AND POTASSIUM FOR FITNESS

Zinc is an essential trace element that is involved in protein, fat, and cell metabolism; it strengthens the immune system and affects insulin production. It is essential for many hormonal functions, including thyroid hormone and testosterone production; testosterone ensures solid connective tissues in both men and women. Zinc also plays a role in wound healing, and exists in the walls of connective tissue cells as well as being an essential component in the synthesis of collagen. A lack of zinc manifests itself through impaired wound healing, weak connective tissues, and general susceptibility to infections. Good sources of zinc are beef and pork, eggs, milk, cheese, legumes, nuts, seafood, and offal. Zinc is absorbed more efficiently from meat and animal products than from vegetables.

Magnesium and potassium also affect cell metabolism and growth, collagen synthesis, and hydration levels; their intake should be adequately monitored. Good sources of magnesium are mineral water, many nuts, and particularly sunflower seeds. Mushrooms, bananas, beans, cheese, spinach, and potatoes are high in potassium.

Incredible sources of zinc are liver, oysters, and shrimps, as well as nuts and meat.

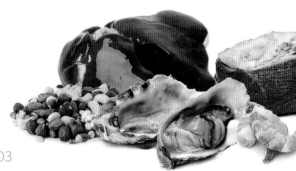

GET ENOUGH SLEEP!

When we sleep, our entire system, but in particular the connective tissues and the intervertebral discs, undergoes a process of regeneration. The intervertebral discs can absorb liquid again, provided they rest long enough so that they are able to soak up fresh nutrients. In addition, only in deep sleep is the human growth hormone (HGH) secreted, which stimulates the synthesis of collagen in the connective tissue cells. Adequate and restful sleep is therefore important. Here are some tips:

● Go to bed at regular times—try not to stay up past your normal bedtime.

● Get enough sleep—for most people this means between seven and nine hours.

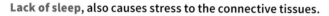

Lack of sleep, also causes stress to the connective tissues.

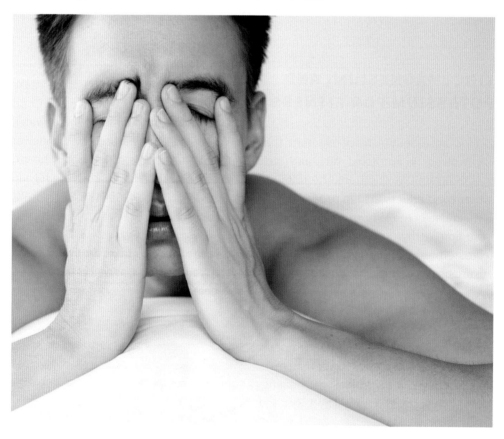

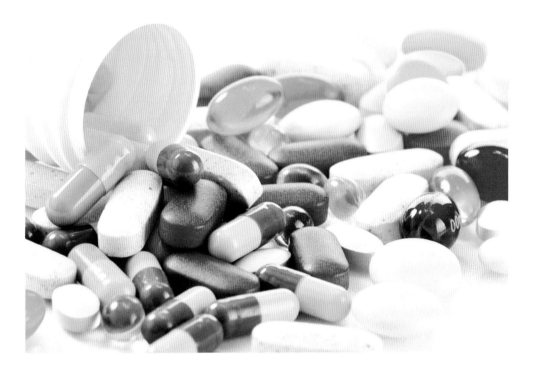

Colourful pills make it seem easy to take vitamins.

● Take breaks during the day, especially at lunchtime. Physiologically, the body is programed to rest at midday, and to slow down. The more you adhere to this rhythm, the less stress you will put on your body.

DO ANY FOOD SUPPLEMENTS MAKE SENSE?

Silica, silicon, vitamin C, zinc, minerals, trace elements, and vitamin B complex are all recommended for the connective tissues. You can simply take a pill, instead of spending time preparing the right food to absorb these vitamins and minerals. However, it is indisputable that vitamins and trace elements are more effective if they enter the body in the form of real food, because it is full of other healthy materials. Natural vitamins are included in sources that are high in roughage, specifically vegetables and fruit, which contain many more secondary plant substances than vitamin and trace element pills alone. Likewise, meat, eggs, and milk provide important fats.

Zinc is a particular exception. It is one of the few trace elements in which there can be a latent deficiency; therefore, the occasional short treatment of zinc tablets will do no harm. Nonetheless, it is wise to seek advice from a pharmacist or a doctor.

B vitamins, of which there are eight in total, belong to those vitamins which you can replenish at any time after infectious diseases, periods of stress, or various diets. They are stored in the body, and the reserves can dwindle at certain times. To top up the storage, it is recommended to take some vitamin B complex, but once again it is wise to seek advice from the doctor or pharmacist.

Silica is a mixture of substances, one of which is silicon. Traditionally, it is considered in alternative therapy circles to be most useful for connective tissue, hair, and nails. Actually, silicon is a component of connective tissue. Whether silica, when taken as a supplement, has the desired effect in terms of enabling the fascia to accumulate it has not been proved. Some time ago, silica products were excluded by some advisers, the reasons being that they contained sand and were dirty, as well as their possibly being linked to kidney damage. The Consumer Council of Hamburg issued a damning verdict after federal and state authorities examined silica products, and doctors vigorously advised against using them.

MY PERSONAL HEALTH ADVICE

From time to time, I take a course of herbal extracts, vitamins, and minerals in small doses, but only for a few weeks of the year, and with breaks. The substances that I use occasionally include zinc and vitamin C, but also curcumin and green tea powder. Curcumin is the main ingredient of the Indian spice turmeric and is used in Ayurvedic medicine as a folk remedy. Modern research has certified that the yellow spice genuinely has an anti-inflammatory effect. Curcumin also has an impact on the growth of certain tumors. It has been confirmed that similar effects occur with green tea powder or green tea: the active ingredients tend to reduce the number of free radicals in the body and are therefore considered anti-inflammatory and preventive in many ways.

Sports physician, and supervisor of the German national football team, Hans-Wilhelm Müller-Wohlfahrt has developed an interesting mixture of ingredients that I would like to try at some point. It contains various vitamins and trace elements, as well as important amino acids, but, to my

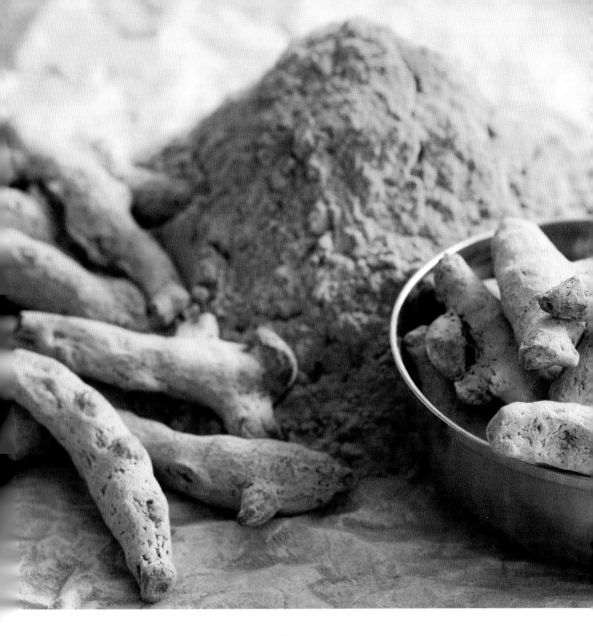

Turmeric contains an anti-inflammatory substance.

knowledge, it is not yet based on robust clinical studies. Nonetheless, even though I prefer to take in all the necessary nutrients only by means of a normal mixed diet, it may be that in exceptional circumstances—for example stress, disease, or competitive sports—such a supplement might prove useful.

The future belongs to the fascia!

Did I manage to inspire you to look further into the fascinating world of fascia and its role in physical health? I hope so, because I am sure that everyone, regardless of age and health, will benefit in everyday life from targeted fascia training and more-creative movement.

If you want to practice in a group rather than alone you can contact the Fitness Fascial Association, which I co-founded. In Germany there are more than 600 qualified fascia trainers who work in their own studios throughout the country. There is an ongoing education program for those interested in training in their own studios throughout Germany, as well as an education program for people who wish to obtain a trainer license.

If you would prefer to practice under supervision in order to learn more about fascia training, you can search for a studio near you. It is important that you have fun in working toward your goal of feeling free and making your movements more elegant and smooth.

Regular group training can be very helpful, along with one-to-one coaching from an experienced Fascial Fitness trainer. This is especially beneficial for beginners and the elderly.

Finally, I would like to take a look into the future. I believe that besides the fascia outlook, there is also a public health perspective to be considered, which we discovered in Chapter 2 with regard to playgrounds for adults. Adults, especially the older generation, should become more versatile and move in a more fascia-friendly and playful manner. This approach can motivate many people in fun and enjoyable ways. Perhaps the trend toward adult playgrounds will inspire their inclusion in general health programs in the future, and communities will provide fascial playgrounds for all generations. This is by no means a utopian fantasy, but a real opportunity for our industrial nations to show more citizens ways of having fun and keeping in good shape. This will help combat joint disease, back pain, arthritis, and obesity—health problems that cost billions every year.

Nowadays, fascia training and objective views of the fascia in sport and medicine are becoming absolutely essential—and this is just the beginning. The fascia research group, myself included, at the University of Ulm are planning scientific studies of the effectiveness of a series of fascial exercises, to be launched in the coming years; these studies will include both sport-related aspects and back pain. The group collaborates with sports scientists from other national and international universities, and we are very excited to learn the outcome of the studies. It will certainly help us to improve our practices and methods; this can be achieved in the fields of various sports and types of training, but especially in the medical sector, more specifically in rehabilitation and prevention.

There are, however, other facets to the future of fascia training. In recent years the body therapist and Fascial Fitness trainer Divo Gitta Müller has developed a special fascia movement program for women, which she offers at her studio in Munich. In addition to addressing muscle stiffening and shortening, a special focus is put on the tonification of tissue areas which are too loose. Not only are the visible and tangible rejuvenation effects of regular exercise physically apparent on the participants: she has revealed that they also recognize a rejuvenating, feel-good effect again in everyday life. For me this is gratifying in a special way, because I have been married to Divo Gitta Müller for 10 years. I would therefore first of all like to thank you, dear Divo, for the many inspiring ideas, for the loving emotional support, and for the many years of fruitful collaboration.

I am also grateful to my team in the Fascia Research Group at the University of Ulm, to my longtime teacher colleagues at the International Rolf Institute in Boulder, Colorado, and to the enthusiastic team of trainers of the Fascial Fitness Association.

I dedicate this book, however, with my special thanks, to my publisher Riva Verlag, who had the idea and, after several attempts, successfully persuaded me to complete this text.

Finally, I would like to give even greater recognition to my co-author, the science journalist Johanna Bayer. Through television reports, she has succeeded in conveying something of the fascination of the recent developments in fascia. She has also professionally and brilliantly taken care of the difficult task of finding the right balance between audience-friendly readability and scientific accuracy.

ADDRESSES · LINKS · INFO

▦ Literature

Müller-Wohlfahrt, Dr. Hans-Wilhelm: *Mensch, beweg dich! So stärken Sie Ihr Bindegewebe*, dtv, München 2004

Myers, Thomas: Anatomy Trains: *Myofascial Meridians for Manual and Movement Therapists*, 3rd edn. Churchill Livingston Elsevier: Edinburgh 2014

Pischinger, Alfred, et al.: *The Extracellular Matrix and Ground Regulation*. North Atlantic Books, Berkeley 2007

Schifter, Roland, and Elke Harms: *Connective Tissue Massage*. Thieme Publishers, Stuttgart 2014

Schleip, Robert, and Baker, Amanda: *Fascia in Sport and Movement*. Handspring Publishing, Edinburgh 2015

Schleip, Robert u.a. (Eds.): *Fascia – the Tensional Network of the Human Body*. Churchill Livingstone, Edinburgh 2012

▦ Links and Addresses

Fascial fitness network, with general information, list of certified trainers, and information about training: **fascial-fitness.de/en/**

Fascial movement program all about harmonious movements, developed by the fascia and body therapist Divo Gitta Müller, Munich [in German]: **bodybliss.de**

Rolf Institute of Structural Integration, with lists of therapists: **rolf.org**

Fascia Research Group page of the University of Ulm: **fasciaresearch.de**

Foam roller for fascia exercises from sports stores, for example: **perform-better.de/en/home**

▦ Companies Who Build or Operate Playgrounds for Adults

USA: aaastateofplay.com

Australia/New Zealand: playgroundcentre.com

Germany: playfit.de/outdoor-fitness.html

Austria: gartenderbewegung.at

ABOUT THE AUTHORS

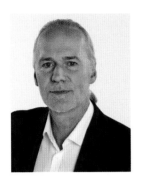

■ Robert Schleip

is regarded as one of the leading experts in the field of fascia research internationally; he holds a doctorate in human biology and is a certified Rolfer as well as a psychologist. As a scientist at the University of Ulm, he leads the Fascia Research Group, and also works as a manual Rolfing therapist at his own private practice. In a teaching capacity, he gives lectures on physiotherapy, osteopathy, and exercise science. He collaborates with scientists and therapists in a global network of research concerning connective tissue.

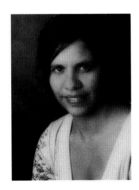

■ Johanna Bayer

is a science journalist and writer for television broadcasting at ARD, WDR, and Arte, and also for consumer magazines. She regularly works on medical topics, including muscles and movement, nutrition, brain research, and anthropology. She has frequently been involved with television programs and press articles regarding the fascia and its implications for training, daily life, and pain.

PICTURE CREDITS

Page 5, 6, 90, 92–96, 104, 106–109, 113, 114 top, 115, 116 top, 117, 119, 120 right, 121, 123, 125, 127–133, 135–137, 138 bottom, 139–150, 151 bottom, 152–156, 159, 161, 163–165, 167–171, 173–175, 177–179, 182–185: ©Vukašin Latinović

Page 4, 6: courtesy of www.eden-reha.de

Page 8: ©fascialnet.com

Page 9, 15 and 211 top: Robert Schleip

Page 10: ©imago/Ulmer

Page 11: courtesy of Endovivo Productions and Dr. J. Guimberteau

Page 13: ©shutterstock/ayakovlevcom

Page 16, 25: ©fascialnet.com

Page 18: ©fotolia/Christian Jung

Page 19: ©ScienceFoto.de/Dr. André Kempe

Page 20, 73 left and right: ©Dr. Christian Schmelzer, Dr. Andrea Heinz, Institut für Angewandte Dermatopharmazie, Martin-Luther-Universität Halle-Wittenberg e.V., Halle (Saale)

Page 21, 55, 61 right, 62, 100–103, 116 bottom, 157: Kristin Hoffmann

Page 23: ©shutterstock/topseller

Page 28: ©fotolia/Cara-Foto

Page 30 right: ©fascialnet.com

Page 30 left bottom: modified image by Nishimura, T. et al. 1994 (*Acta Anat* 151: 250–257), courtesy of Karger Publishers

Page 31: ©fotolia/adimas

Page 34, 37, 39, 40, 43: Laura Osswald

Page 38, 194: ©European Rolfing Association e.V.

Page 45: shutterstock/snapgalleria

Page 46: ©shutterstock/Andrey_Popov

Page 48, 68 left top: Tittel, K. 2012 (*Beschreibende und funktionelle Anatomie*, 15th edn, Kiener Verlag, Munich: 273)

Page 49: picture-alliance/united archives

Page 50: ©shutterstock/Lucky Business

Page 51: ©shutterstock/Vadim Georgiev

Page 52: ©shutterstock/8th.creator

Page 53: Kristin Hoffmann, using an image from shutterstock/stihii

Page 54: Kristin Hoffmann, after an illustration from Rode, C. 2010 ("Interaction between passive and contractile muscle elements: Re-evaluation and new mechanisms, Ph.D. thesis," Jena, Germany). See: http://wiki.ifs-tud. de/_media/biomechanik/projekte/interaktion_zwischen_passiven_und_kontraktilen_muskelelementen_ neubewertung_und_neue_mechanismen_von_dr._christian_rode.pdf, based on an illustration from Hill, A.V. 1938 ("The heat of shortening and the dynamic constants of muscle," *Proc Royal Soc London: Series B*: 126, 136–195)

Page 56 top left: ©fotolia/JohanSwanepoel

Page 56 top right: ©shutterstock/dlodewijks

Page 56 bottom: ©shutterstock/Christopher Meder

Page 57: ©shutterstock/Stephen Coburn

Page 59: ©shutterstock/SJ Allen

Page 60: ©fotolia/takasu

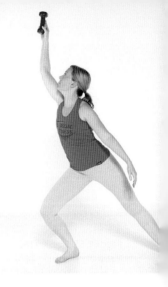

EXERCISE OVERVIEW

Basic Program 112–125
    Rolling Out the Feet 114
    Calves and Achilles Tendon: Elastic Jumps 116
    Front and Rear Line Stretches: Eagle Flight 118
    Waist and Side Stretches: Eagle Wings on a Chair 120
    Shoulder and Shoulder Girdle Activation: Spring-Backs Against A Wall 122
    Neck and Back Relaxation: Snake Dance 124

Exercises for Problem Areas: Back, Neck, Arms, Hips, Feet.................................... 126–156
   Short Back Program 127–137
    Rolling Out the Lumbar Fascia 128
    Back Stretch: the Cat 130
    African Bends 132
    Flying Sword 134
    Verebral Chain Relief 136
   At the Office: Problems in the Neck, Arms, and Shoulders 138–143
    Shoulder Stretch 139
    Freedom for the Neck 140
    Relaxation for Tired Forearms 141
    Momentum for the Whole Body: Swinging Bamboo 142
   Around the Hips... 144–150
    Rolling Out the Thigh 145
    Activating the Outer Thigh 146
    Swinging the Legs 148
    The Skate 150
   For the Feet and Stance 151–156
    Rolling Out the Plantar Fascia 152
    Sensitizing the Soles of the Feet 152
    Swinging the Legs 154
    Elastic Jumping for the Feet, Calves, and Achilles Tendon 155
    Stretching the Achilles Tendon 156

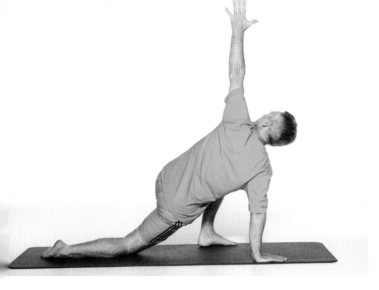

INDEX

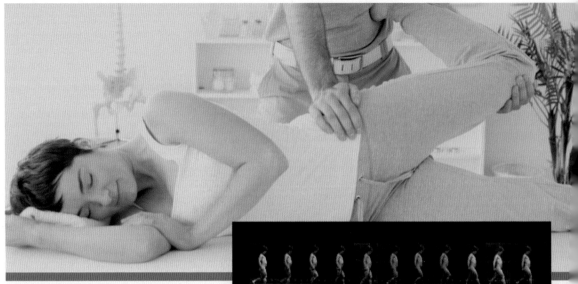
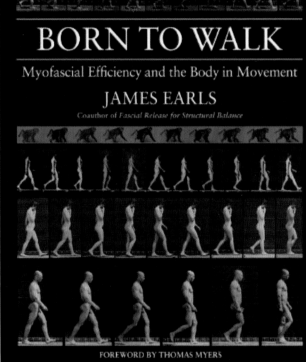